POCKET GUIDE TO

Pediatric Nutrition Assessment

THIRD EDITION

Beth Leonberg

MS, MA, RDN, CSP, LDN, FAND

Academy of Nutrition and Dietetics
Chicago, IL

eat right. Academy of Nutrition and Dietetics

Academy of Nutrition and Dietetics
120 S. Riverside Plaza, Suite 2190
Chicago, IL 60606

Academy of Nutrition and Dietetics Pocket Guide to Pediatric Nutrition Assessment, Third Edition

ISBN 978-0-88091-010-1 (print)
ISBN 978-0-88091-015-6 (eBook)
Catalog Number 367320 (print)
Catalog Number 367320e (eBook)

10   9   8   7   6   5   4   3   2   1

For more information on the Academy of Nutrition and Dietetics, visit www.eatright.org

Library of Congress Cataloging-in-Publication Data

Names: Leonberg, Beth L., author.
Title: Pocket guide to pediatric nutrition assessment / Beth Leonberg, MS, MA, RDN, CSP, LDN, FAND.
Description: Third edition. | Chicago, IL : Academy of Nutrition and Dietetics, [2020] | Includes bibliographical references and index. | Summary: "This comprehensive, easy-to-navigate guide has been updated to include information on the use of CDC, WHO, and specialized growth charts; vitamin D recommendations; and screening information. It also features expanded, easier-to-read coverage of laboratory tests and nutrient needs. An essential tool for any RDN who provides nutrition care to pediatric patients!"-- Provided by publisher.
Identifiers: LCCN 2019027585 (print) | LCCN 2019027586 (ebook) | ISBN 9780880910101 (print) | ISBN 9780880910156 (ebook)
Subjects: LCSH: Children--Nutrition--Handbooks, manuals, etc.
Classification: LCC RJ206 .L37 2020 (print) | LCC RJ206 (ebook) | DDC 618.92--dc23
LC record available at https://lccn.loc.gov/2019027585
LC ebook record available at https://lccn.loc.gov/2019027586

Contents

List of Boxes and Tables

Boxes

Tables

Frequently Used Terms/Abbreviations

AAP	American Academy of Pediatrics
AI	adequate intake
AMA	American Medical Association
ASPEN	American Society for Parenteral and Enteral Nutrition
BMI	body mass index
BMR	basal metabolic rate
CDC	Centers for Disease Control and Prevention
CPE	Continuing Professional Education
DRI	Dietary Reference Intake
EAR	Estimated Average Requirement
EER	Estimated Energy Requirement

eNCPT	electronic Nutrition Care Process Terminology
Hct	hematocrit
Hgb	hemoglobin
INTER-GROWTH-21st	International Fetal and Newborn Growth Consortium for the 21st Century
MCV	mean cell volume
MUAC	mid–upper arm circumference
NCP	Nutrition Care Process
NFPE	nutrition-focused physical examination
NHANES	National Health and Nutrition Examination Survey
NRST-CF	Nutrition Risk Screening Tool for Children and Adolescents with Cystic Fibrosis
NutriSTEP	Nutrition Screening for Toddlers and Preschoolers
OFC	occipital frontal circumference
PAL	physical activity level

PeDiSMART	Pediatric Digital Scaled Malnutrition Risk Screening Tool
PNST	Pediatric Nutrition Screening Tool
PYMS	Paediatric Yorkhill Malnutrition Score
RDA	Recommended Dietary Allowance
REE	Resting Energy Expenditure
RQ	respiratory quotient
SAM	severe acute malnutrition
SAS	Statistical Analysis System
SDs	standard deviations
SGNA	Subjective Global Nutritional Assessment
STAMP	Screening Tool for the Assessment of Malnutrition in Paediatrics
STRONGkids	Screening Tool for Risk on Nutritional Status and Growth
TEE	total energy expenditure
TIBC	total iron-binding capacity
TSF	triceps skinfold

UL	Tolerable Upper Intake Level
UNICEF	United Nations Children's Fund
USDA	US Department of Agriculture
WHO	World Health Organization
WIC	Women, Infants, and Children

Reviewers

Aida Miles, MMSc, RDN, LD, LMNT, FAND
Director, Coordinated MPH Nutrition Program,
University of Minnesota, School of Public Health
Minneapolis, MN

Nancy Nevin-Folino, RDN, LD, FADA, FAND
Neonatal Nutrition Support Specialist, Dayton
Children's Hospital
Dayton, OH

Beth Ogata, MS, RDN, CSP
Lecturer, University of Washington, Center on
Human Development and Disability
Seattle, WA

Sandra Robbins, RDN, CSP
Nutritionist, Pediatric Lung and Allergy Center
Fairfax, VA

Bonnie A. Spear, PhD, RDN, FAND
Professor Pediatrics Emerita, University of Alabama—
Birmingham
Birmingham, AL

Jodi Wolff, MS, RDN, LD, FAND, FAACPDM
Pediatric Dietitian, Rainbow Babies Children's
Hospital
Solon, OH

Preface

The challenge of accurately assessing and diagnosing pediatric nutrition problems is endlessly fascinating to clinicians and is critical to helping families care for their children. While some children present with a constellation of concerns that seem familiar and easy to address, there is virtually always a unique twist that makes each child's nutrition problem an individual puzzle to put together. Assessing each domain of nutrition information is necessary to bring the puzzle into focus.

Understanding of how to assess, interpret, and communicate each piece of the assessment puzzle continues to evolve. This evolution sometimes leads us to circle back again to our most basic ways of defining and describing nutrition risk. Over the past decade, experts have revisited the concept of pediatric malnutrition, resulting in new ways of assessing and classifying it. This third edition of the *Pocket Guide to Pediatric Nutrition Assessment* includes updated recommendations based on the latest expert guidelines published by the Academy of Nutrition and Dietetics, the American Society for Parenteral and Enteral Nutrition (ASPEN), and the World Health Organization (WHO). The list below provides a brief overview of what is new in the third edition:

Chapter 1:
- Updated and expanded description of nutrition assessment as the first step of the Nutrition Care Process

Chapter 2:
- Academy of Nutrition and Dietetics/ASPEN indicators of pediatric malnutrition (undernutrition)
- Summary and discussion of validated pediatric malnutrition risk screening tools

Chapter 3:
- Updated and expanded list of specialized growth charts
- Discussion of z scores
- Table of resources for determining anthropometric z scores
- Expanded discussion of mid–upper arm circumference and addition of percentile tables
- WHO and UNICEF definition of severe acute malnutrition
- Academy of Nutrition and Dietetics/ASPEN criteria to identify and classify degree of malnutrition

Chapter 5:

- Updated baby foods
- Updated tables of amounts needed from each food group to meet calorie levels recommended by the US Department of Health and Human Services and the US Department of Agriculture in the *2015–2020 Dietary Guidelines for Americans* and MyPlate

Chapter 6:

- Updated and expanded information on pediatric nutrition–focused physical exam

Chapter 8:

- Inclusion of key Dietary Reference Intake (DRI) values
- Sample calculation for estimating energy needs using the Estimated Energy Requirement (EER) equations
- Basal metabolic rate (BMR) prediction equations for obese children and adolescents
- Updated references for nutrients of special concern

The goal is for this pocket guide to support practitioners in putting together the pieces of the nutrition assessment puzzle for each child assessed, using the most current tools and language.

Beth L. Leonberg, MS, MA, RDN, CSP, LDN, FAND

CHAPTER 1

Nutrition Care Process

The Nutrition Care Process (NCP) is designed to improve the quality and consistency of patient/client care and the resulting patient/client outcomes. The emphasis is on standardizing the *care process*, rather than standardizing individual patient/client care.[1,2] This chapter provides an overview of the four steps of the NCP (see Box 1.1 on page 2) and sets the context for the rest of the pocket guide, which focuses on the first step of the NCP, nutrition assessment. Screening for nutrition risk is an additional step that precedes the NCP and will be discussed in detail in Chapter 2.

BOX 1.1   Steps in the Nutrition Care Process[1,2]

Step 1: Nutrition Assessment

A method for obtaining, verifying, interpreting, and documenting data needed to identify a nutrition-related problem.

Step 2: Nutrition Diagnosis

The identification and labeling of a specific nutrition problem that a dietetics practitioner is responsible for treating independently. Nutrition diagnoses may be temporary and resolved with nutrition interventions, as opposed to medical diagnoses, which pertain to diseases or pathologies of organs or body systems. This step results in the documentation of the nutrition diagnosis (PES) statement, which is composed of the following components: the problem (P), the etiology (E), and the signs and symptoms (S).

Step 3: Nutrition Intervention

Specific actions taken to change nutrition-related behaviors, risk factors, environmental conditions, or aspects of nutritional health.

Step 4: Nutrition Monitoring and Evaluation

The review of the patient/client's status at a preplanned follow-up and the systematic comparison of current findings with previous status, intervention goals, or a reference standard.

Box 1.2 outlines the characteristics of the first step of the process, nutrition assessment or reassessment. Included within this framework are critical thinking skills essential to the nutrition assessment process, which were outlined in the Academy of Nutrition and Dietetics practice paper Critical Thinking Skills in Nutrition Assessment and Diagnosis.[3] Dietetics practitioners are encouraged to develop and advance their critical thinking skills over the span of their career in order to provide accurate and comprehensive nutrition assessment and reassessment. Standardized terminology used in documenting the NCP is available electronically in the electronic Nutrition Care Process Terminology (eNCPT).[4]

BOX 1.2   Step 1: Nutrition Assessment and Reassessment

Definition and purpose

Nutrition assessment is a systematic approach to collect, classify, and synthesize important and relevant data from clients (where *clients* refers to individuals and population). This step also includes reassessment, which additionally includes collection of new data and comparing and reevaluating data from the previous interaction to the next. Nutrition assessment is an ongoing, dynamic process that involves initial data collection as well as continual reassessment and analysis of the client's status compared with accepted standards, recommendations, or goals.

Continued on next page

BOX 1.2   Step 1: Nutrition Assessment and Reassessment (cont.)

Data sources/tools for assessment

Screening or referral form

Client interview

Medical or health records

Consultation with other caregivers, including family members

Community-based surveys and focus groups

Statistical reports, administrative data, and epidemiologic studies

Types of data collected

Food- and nutrition-related history

Anthropometric measurements

Biochemical data, medical tests, and procedures

Nutrition-focused physical examination findings

Client history

Nutrition assessment components

Review data collected for factors that affect nutrition and health status.

Cluster individual data to identify at least one nutrition diagnosis as described in diagnosis reference sheets.

Identify accepted standards, recommendations, and/or goals by which data will be compared.

**BOX 1.2   Step 1: Nutrition Assessment and
Reassessment (cont.)**

Reassessment components

Collect new data.

Compare data with previous interaction(s).

Compare the monitoring and evaluation outcomes/indicators
documented in the previous interaction to the new data.

Evaluate if the client's nutritional status has changed to
demonstrate effectiveness of intervention.

Evaluate the status of the nutrition diagnosis.

Evaluate whether the nutrition assessment data from the
previous interaction need to be reassessed or changed
depending on the client's status or situation.

Identify new nutrition assessment data to monitor and evaluate during the next interaction.

Critical thinking

Determining important and relevant data to collect

Determining the need for additional information

Selecting assessment tools and procedures that match
the situation

Applying assessment tools in valid and reliable ways

Validating the data

Continued on next page

BOX 1.2   Step 1: Nutrition Assessment and Reassessment (cont.)

Determination for continuation of care

If upon completion of an initial nutrition assessment or reassessment it is determined that the problem cannot be modified by further nutrition care, discharge or discontinuation from this episode of nutrition care may be appropriate.

Adapted with permission from Swan WI, Vivanti A, Hakel-Smith NA, et al. Nutrition Care Process and Model Update: toward realizing people-centered care and outcomes management. *J Acad Nutr Diet.* 2017;117(12):2003-2014.[1]

References

1. Swan WI, Vivanti A, Hakel-Smith NA, et al. Nutrition Care Process and Model Update: toward realizing people-centered care and outcomes management. *J Acad Nutr Diet.* 2017;117(12):2003-2014.

2. Academy of Nutrition and Dietetics. *Abridged Nutrition Care Process Terminology (NCPT) Reference Manual: Standardized Terminology for the Nutrition Care Process.* Chicago, IL: Academy of Nutrition and Dietetics; 2017.

3. Charney P, Peterson SJ. Practice Paper of the Academy of Nutrition and Dietetics: critical thinking skills in nutrition assessment and diagnosis. *J Acad Nutr Diet.* 2013;113(11):1545.

4. Academy of Nutrition and Dietetics. Nutrition Terminology Reference Manual (eNCPT): Dietetics Language for Nutrition Care. www.ncpro.org. Accessed May 16, 2019.

CHAPTER 2

Nutrition Risk Screening

The purpose of nutrition screening is to identify individuals at risk for nutrition problems who will benefit from a more complete assessment and development of a nutrition care plan via the Nutrition Care Process (NCP).[1] Although not part of the NCP, screening is nevertheless important to the process because it identifies clients who would benefit from nutrition care or medical nutrition therapy. Within the pediatric population, use of a standard screening tool was shown to improve compliance with measurement of anthropometrics on admission to the hospital.[2]

Certain characteristics should be taken into consideration when developing and conducting a nutrition risk screen. Screening should be cost-effective, involve minimal risk for the person being screened, use readily available data, and use the fewest resources necessary to accomplish the goal. Effective screening must also be accurate, which is defined by:

- sensitivity—the ability to identify all those at risk;
- specificity—the ability to identify all those not at risk; and
- positive and negative predictive value—that is, a high likelihood that a subject who is identified as "at risk" actually is at risk and a low likelihood that a subject who is not identified as at risk truly is at risk.[3]

Finally, screening is effective only if it can lead to interventions that increase the likelihood of positive health outcomes.

Screening Parameters and Assignment of Risk

Screening for nutrition risk involves the comparison of a set of parameters, such as anthropometric indicators, dietary intake, or biochemical data, against standards that identify nutrition risk. Five key areas for assessment when identifying pediatric malnutrition were defined by Mehta and colleagues in a landmark article published in 2013.[4] The five domains include the following: anthropometric variables, growth, chronicity of malnutrition, etiology of malnutrition and etiology of pathogenesis, and impact of malnutrition on functional status.

A screen may be designed broadly to identify many individuals with a range of nutrition-related risk factors. For example, a nutrition screening may be performed on all patients at the time of admission to acute care facilities. A screen may also be designed more narrowly to identify only those with selected nutritional risk factors (eg, those at risk of insufficient intake of a particular nutrient in a public health setting), or to identify specific levels of nutrition risk. Within groups of children with the same medical diagnosis (eg, children with cystic fibrosis or cancer) screening can be used to predict outcomes and to identify those with the greatest need for intervention.[5,6] Although each facility must define risk and establish policies and procedures appropriate to its setting and client population, the recent development of a multitude of pediatric malnutrition screening tools points to the goal of identifying a more universal language and methodology for describing malnutrition.[7-16] See Box 2.1 (pages 10 and 11) for a list of typical parameters that may be used in pediatric nutrition risk screening.

BOX 2.1   Typical Parameters That *May* Be Used to Determine Nutritional Risk

Anthropometrics[a]
Weight-for-age (< or > selected percentile)

Length/height-for-age (< selected percentile)

Weight-for-length/height (< or > selected percentile)

Head circumference-for-age (< selected percentile)

Body mass index-for-age (>85th percentile)

Changes in rate of weight gain or growth

Percentage of 50th-percentile-weight for height

Classification of stunting or wasting by accepted standards

Client History
Anemia

Anorexia nervosa, bulimia nervosa, or other eating disorder

Bone marrow transplant

Bronchopulmonary dysplasia

Burns

Cancer

Cardiac disease

Cystic fibrosis

Developmental disabilities

Diabetes

Failure to thrive/malnutrition

Gastrointestinal disorder (inflammatory bowel disease, malabsorption, short bowel syndrome, vomiting, or diarrhea)

BOX 2.1   Typical Parameters That *May* Be Used to Determine Nutritional Risk (cont.)

HIV and AIDS

Inborn errors of metabolism

Liver disease

Overweight, at risk of overweight, or obesity

Pregnancy

Prematurity or low birth weight

Renal disease

Rickets

Seizure disorder

Sepsis, severe

Ventilator dependency

Medications that interact with foods or nutrients

Food and Nutrition History

Special/modified diet order (eg, nil per os, clear liquid)

Enteral nutrition support

Parenteral nutrition support

Food allergies or intolerances

Biochemical Data

Hemoglobin/hematocrit

Total lymphocyte count

Albumin/prealbumin

[a] Evaluated using age-specific (or corrected age for premature infants) and gender-specific standards.

Screening Tools and Personnel

Nutrition risk screening tools are often designed to assign points for each risk factor; the highest cumulative point value indicates the greatest nutrition risk and results in the most immediate or extensive intervention. Alternatively, screening may result in a simple classification of risk or no risk (without any ranking order).

The screening process itself can be completed by a nutrition and dietetics technician, registered, a registered dietitian nutritionist, other food and nutrition services personnel, or any other qualified member of the health care team, such as a nurse or physician. Screening may be conducted through an in-person interview, through a manual review of the medical record, or with a computerized algorithm. In the past, inpatient nutrition screening was routinely done on a manual basis using a unique form designed to capture and evaluate parameters. However, hospital-based nutrition screening is now more often part of the electronic medical record and may be integrated into the multidisciplinary admission database. Screening in ambulatory and community settings may still be conducted manually.

Screening in Clinical Settings

Nutrition risk screening may occur in many clinical settings, such as:

- acute care hospitals,
- home care agencies,

- ambulatory care centers, and
- physician offices.

Joint Commission Requirements

Although the Joint Commission has previously required that nutritional screening be performed within 24 hours after inpatient admission, the most recent standards are less prescriptive.[17] Health care organizations are required to set appropriate standards for assessment and reassessment of patients and to document them in writing. Among the Elements of Performance in Standard PC.01.02.01 is the following statement: "The hospital has defined criteria that identify when nutritional plans are developed."

American Society for Parenteral and Enteral Nutrition Standards

The American Society for Parenteral and Enteral Nutrition (ASPEN) has similarly established standards related to screening for nutrition risk in hospitalized pediatric patients. See Box 2.2 on page 14.

> **BOX 2.2   American Society for Parenteral and Enteral
> Nutrition (ASPEN) Standards for Nutrition
> Support: Hospitalized Pediatric Patients**
>
> **Standard 4. Nutrition Screening**
> **4.1:** The policy and procedure for nutrition screening shall be
> formalized and documented.
>
> **4.1.1** All patients shall be screened for nutrition risk
> within 24 hours after admission.
>
> **4.1.2** The result of the nutrition screen shall be docu-
> mented and appropriate intervention initiated.
>
> **4.1.3** A procedure for nutrition rescreening should be
> implemented.

Adapted with permission from Wiley & Sons, Inc. Corkins MR, Griggs KC, Groh-Wargo S, et al; Task Force on Standards for Nutrition Support: Pediatric Hospitalized Patients, American Society for Parenteral and Enteral Nutrition Board of Directors. Standards for nutrition support: pediatric hospitalized patients. *Nutr Clin Pract.* 2013;28:263-276.[18]

Screening the Hospitalized Patient

Over the last decade, a number of different pediatric nutrition risk screening tools have been developed to identify malnutrition in hospitalized infants and children.[8-16] Table 2.1 provides a brief description of these tools.

TABLE 2.1 Pediatric Nutrition Risk Screening Tools[8-16]

Tool	Screening Parameters	Population Characteristics	Sensitivity	Specificity	Positive/Negative Predictive Value	Agreement with Other Tools
Screening Tool for the Assessment of Malnutrition in Paediatrics (STAMP)[10]	Weight <2nd or >98th percentile; parent reported weight loss in last month; parent reported irregular meals; and parent reported reduced appetite	122 children, mean age 8.2–8.4 y Target population: hospitalized children 2–17 y	70%	91%	55%	
Subjective Global Nutritional Assessment (SGNA)[11,12]	Insufficient food intake; weight loss over time; loss of muscle mass; loss of fat mass; fluid accumulation; and diminished grip strength	150 children, mean age 23 mo	Not reported	Not reported		Moderate-to-strong correlation with anthropometric measures

Continued on next page

TABLE 2.1 Pediatric Nutrition Risk Screening Tools[8-16] (cont.)

Tool	Screening Parameters	Population Characteristics	Sensitivity	Specificity	Positive/Negative Predictive Value	Agreement with Other Tools
Paediatric Yorkhill Malnutrition Score (PYMS)[8,9]	Body mass index (BMI); recent weight loss; decreased intake ≥ 1 wk; and anticipated impact of illness/admission on nutritional status	1,571 children: 1,208 in tertiary pediatric hospital, median age 6.3 y; 363 in community hospital, median age 7.6 y	59%	92%	47%	80% with STAMP; 81% with SGNA
Screening Tool for Risk on Nutritional Status and Growth (STRONGkids)[13,14]	Subjective clinical assessment; high-risk disease; nutritional intake; and weight loss	424 children, median age 3.5 y	71.9%	49.1%	11.9%	

Tool	Criteria	Population				
Pediatric Digital Scaled Malnutrition Risk screening Tool (PeDiSMART)[15]	Weight-for-age z score; nutrition intake level; overall disease impact; and symptoms affecting intake	500 children, median age 2.4 y. Target population: patients 1 mo to 17 y	87% for detecting weight loss/ nutrition support	75% for detecting weight loss/ nutrition support		
Pediatric Nutrition Screening Tool (PNST)[16]	Unintentional weight loss; poor weight gain over last few months; eating/feeding less in last few weeks; obviously underweight/ significantly overweight	295 children, median age 10.9 mo	89% for detecting BMI z score ≤ -2	66% for detecting BMI z score ≤ -2	22%/98%	Highly correlated with pediatric SGNA

While Screening Tool for Risk on Nutritional Status and Growth (STRONGkids) was found to be the most reliable in identifying children at nutrition risk in one trial and a systematic review,[19,20] other investigators have endorsed Paediatric Yorkhill Malnutrition Score (PYMS) as the most reliable screening tool.[21] Still other trials[22-24] and a meta-analysis[25] comparing results using more than one of these screening tools have demonstrated that there is poor agreement between the tools and that none is superior to the others. The Academy of Nutrition and Dietetics Evidence Analysis Library recently conducted a systematic review to determine which nutrition screening tools were the most valid and reliable for identifying malnutrition risk in the pediatric population. Thirteen nutrition screening tools examined in 29 studies were included in the systemic review. Nutrition screening tools with Good/Strong or Fair evidence and moderate validity included Screening Tool for the Assessment of Malnutrition in Paediatrics (STAMP), STRONGkids and PYMS in the inpatient setting and Nutrition Risk Screening Tool for Children and Adolescents with Cystic Fibrosis (NRST-CF) in the specialty setting. No tools in the community setting met these criteria. Limitations included few studies examining each tool, heterogeneity between studies examining a common tool, and lack of tools that included currently recommended indicators to identify pediatric malnutrition.[26] Clearly, more research needs to be done to identify one or more tools that are sensitive, specific, and reliable.

Screening for Specialized Patient Populations

The efficacy of malnutrition screening tools has been explored in patients with chronic diseases and conditions with mixed results.[27-31] The following tools have been identified for the populations noted:

- spinal cord injuries—STAMP[28]
- acute burn injuries—STRONGkids, PYMS, and STAMP[29]
- liver disease—STRONGkids[30]
- cerebral palsy—Subjective Global Nutritional Assessment (SGNA)[31]

In addition to applying these more general pediatric screening tools, disease-specific screening tools have been developed to try to identify patients within the population who would benefit most from nutrition assessment and intervention. These tools include the following patient diseases or conditions:

- cystic fibrosis[5,32]
- cancer[6]

Nutrition risk indicators for a wide range of diseases/conditions are identified in the Academy of Nutrition and Dietetics Pediatric Nutrition Care Manual.[33]

Screening in Ambulatory, Community, and Public Health Settings

While the screening of hospitalized pediatric patients has received much attention recently, screening tools for use in ambulatory settings are far fewer. Nutrition risk screening tools for well-child care are available from *Bright Futures Nutrition*, third edition.[34] The Nutrition Screening for Toddlers and Preschoolers (NutriSTEP) was developed as a tool to screen for nutrition risk initially among preschoolers (aged 3 to 5 years)[35] and later modified for use with toddlers (aged 18 to 35 months).[36] Unlike the tools developed for use in the hospital, these tools are parent-administered questionnaires, built upon parents' responses to 17 questions related to growth, food and fluid intake, food group intake, physical activity, and sedentary behaviors. Validation of these instruments demonstrated their sensitivity and specificity when compared to assessment of risk by a registered dietitian nutritionist, showing them to be both reliable and valid.[35,36] At least one study has demonstrated the validity of a modified version of STAMP in an ambulatory setting, allowing for administration of the same tool across settings.[37] More work needs to be done to develop and validate screening tools for ambulatory settings.

Nutrition risk screening in community/public health settings is an important way to identify and prioritize clients in need of further intervention. Nutrition risk screening is a primary function of the nutritionist in the Special Supplemental Nutrition Program for Women, Infants, and Children (WIC). All applicants for WIC are screened for risk, including growth and dietary assessments, and must have either a medical- or dietary-based condition to participate.[38] Other community/public health settings where nutrition risk screening may occur include the following:

- newborn and well-baby clinics
- shelters for women who have experienced domestic abuse or for homeless people
- community or migrant health centers
- early intervention programs
- child-care programs
- schools

References

1. Huysentruyt K, Vandenplas Y, De Schepper J. Screening and assessment tools for pediatric malnutrition. *Curr Opin Clin Nutr Metab Care.* 2016;19:336-340.

2. Milani S, Wright C, Purcell O, Macleod I, Gerasimidis K. Acquisition and utilisation of anthropometric measurement on admission in a paediatric hospital before and after the introduction of a malnutrition screening tool. *J Hum Nutr Diet.* 2013;26:294-297.

3. Field LB, Hand RK. Differentiating malnutrition *screening* and *assessment:* a Nutrition Care Process perspective. *J Acad Nutr Diet.* 2015;115:824-828.

4. Mehta NM, Corkins MR, Lyman B, et al; American Society for Parenteral and Enteral Nutrition Board of Directors. Defining pediatric malnutrition: a paradigm shift toward etiology-related definitions. *J Parenter Enteral Nutr.* 2013;37:460-481.

5. McDonald CM. Validation of a nutrition risk screening tool for children and adolescents with cystic fibrosis ages 2-20 years. *J Ped Gastro Nutr.* 2008;46:438-446.

6. Murphy AJ, White M, Viani K, Mosby TT. Evaluation of the nutrition screening tool for childhood cancer (SCAN). *Clin Nutr.* 2016;35:219-224.

7. Becker P, Carney LN, Corkins MR, et al; Academy of Nutrition and Dietetics, American Society for Parenteral and Enteral Nutrition. Consensus Statement of the Academy of Nutrition and Dietetics/American Society for Parenteral and Enteral Nutrition: indicators recommended for the identification and documentation of pediatric malnutrition (undernutrition). *Nutr Clin Pract.* 2015;30:147-161.

8. Gerasimidis K, Keane O, Macleod I, Flynn DM, Wright CM. A four-stage evaluation of the Paediatric Yorkhill Malnutrition Score in a tertiary paediatric hospital and district general hospital. *Brit J Nutr.* 2010;104:751-756.

9. Gerasimidis K, Macleod I, Maclean A, et al. Performance of the novel Paediatric Yorkhill Malnutrition Score (PYMS) in hospital practice. *Clin Nutr.* 2011;30:430-435.

10. McCarthy H, Dixon M, Crabtree I, Eaton-Evans MJ, McNulty H. The development and evaluation of the Screening Tool for the Assessment of Malnutrition in Paediatrics (STAMP^C) for use by healthcare staff. *J Hum Nutr Diet.* 2012;25:311-318.

11. Secker DJ, Jeejeebhoy KN. How to perform Subjective Global Nutrition Assessment in children. *J Acad Nutr Diet.* 2012;112:424-431.

12. Vermilyea S, Slicker J, El-Chammas K, et al. Subjective Global Nutrition Assessment in critically ill children. *J Parenter Enteral Nutr.* 2013;37:659-666.

13. Hulst JM, Zwart H, Hop WC, Joosten KFM. Dutch national survey to test the STRONGkids nutritional risk screening tool in hospitalized children. *Clin Nutr.* 2010;29:106-111.

14. Huysentruyt K, Alliet P, Muyshont L, et al. The STRONGkids nutritional screening tool in hospitalized children: a validation study. *Nutrition.* 2013;29;1356-1361.

15. Karagiozoglou-Lampoudi T, Daskalou E, Lampoudis D, Apostolou A, Agakidis C. Computer-based malnutrition risk calculations may enhance the ability to identify pediatric patients at malnutrition risk for unfavorable outcome. *J Parenter Enteral Nutr.* 2015;39:418-425.

16. White M, Lawson K, Ramsey R, et al. Simple nutrition screening tool for pediatric inpatients. *J Parenter Enteral Nutr.* 2016;40:392-398.

17. The Joint Commission. 2019 Hospital Accreditation Standards, E-edition. https://e-dition.jcrinc.com /MainContent.aspx. Accessed November 11, 2018.

18. Corkins MR, Griggs KC, Groh-Wargo S, et al; Task Force on Standards for Nutrition Support: Pediatric Hospitalized Patients, American Society for Parenteral and Enteral Nutrition Board of Directors. Standards for nutrition support: pediatric hospitalized patients. *Nutr Clin Pract.* 2013;28:263-276.

19. Moeeni V, Walls T, Day AS. Nutritional status and nutrition risk screening in hospitalized children in New Zealand. *Acta Pediatr.* 2013;102:e419-e423.

20. Teixeira AF, Viana KDAL. Nutritional screening in hospitalized pediatric patients: a systematic review. *J Pediatr (Rio J).* 2016;92:343-352.

21. Wonoputri N, Djais JTB, Rosalina I. Validity of nutritional screening tools for hospitalized children. *J Nutr Metab.* 2014;2014:1-5.

22. Thomas PC, Marino LV, Williams SA, Beattie RM. Outcome of nutritional screening in the acute paediatric setting. *Arch Dis Child.* 2016;101:1119-1124.

23. Chourdakis M, Hecht C, Gerasimidis K, et al. Malnutrition risk in hospitalized children: use of 3 screening tools in a large European population. *Am J Clin Nutr.* 2016;103:1301-1310.

24. Daskalou E, Galli-Tsinopoulou A, Karagiozoglou-Lampoudi T, Augoustides-Savvopoulou P. Malnutrition in hospitalized pediatric patients: assessment, prevalence, and association to adverse outcomes. *J Amer Coll Nutr.* 2016;35:372-380.

25. Huysentruyt K, Devreker T, Dejonckheere J, De Schepper J, Vandenplas Y, Cools F. Accuracy of nutritional screening tools in assessing the risk of undernutrition in hospitalized children. *J Pediatr Gastroenterol Nutr.* 2015;61:159-166.

26. Academy of Nutrition and Dietetics Evidence Analysis Library. Nutrition Screening Pediatrics. www.andeal.org /topic.cfm?menu=5767. Accessed 19 November, 2018.

27. Wiskin AE, Owens DR, Cornelius VR, Wootton SA, Beattie RM. Paediatric nutrition risk scores in clinical practice: children with inflammatory bowel disease. *J Hum Nutr Diet.* 2012;25:319-322.

28. Wong S, Graham A, Hirani SP, Grimble G, Forbes A. Validation of the Screening Tool for the Assessment of Malnutrition in Paediatrics (STAMP) in patients with spinal cord injuries (SCIs). *Spinal Cord.* 2014;51:424-429.

29. Bang YK, Park MK, Ju YS, Cho KY. Clinical significance of
     nutritional risk screening tool for hospitalized children with
     acute burn injuries: a cross-sectional study. *J Hum Nutr Diet.*
     2018;31(3):370-378. doi:10.1111/jhn.12518.

30. Song T, Mu Y, Gong X, Ma W, Li L. Screening for nutritional
     risk in hospitalized children with liver disease. *Asia Pac J Clin
     Nutr.* 2017;25:1107-1112.

31. Minocha P, Sitaraman S, Choudhary A, Yadav R. Subjective
     Global Nutritional Assessment: a reliable screening tool for
     nutritional assessment in Cerebral Palsy Children. *Indian
     J Pediatr.* 2018;85:15-19.

32. Simon MISdS, Forte GC, Pereira JdS, Procianoy EdFA,
     Drehmer M. Validation of a nutrition screening tool for
     pediatric patients with cystic fibrosis. *J Acad Nutr Diet.*
     2016;116:813-818.

33. Academy of Nutrition and Dietetics. Pediatric Nutrition Care
     Manual. www.nutritioncaremanual.org. Accessed January 4,
     2018.

34. The American Academy of Pediatrics. *Bright Futures Nutrition.*
     3rd ed. In: Holt K, Wooldridge N, Story M, Sofka D, eds.
     Washington, DC: The American Academy of Pediatrics; 2011.
     https://brightfutures.aap.org/materials-and-tools/nutrition
     -and-pocket-guide/Pages/default.aspx. Accessed May 16,
     2019.

35. Randall Simpson JA, Keller HH, Rysdale LA, Beyers JE.
     Nutrition Screening Tool for Every Preschooler (NutriSTEP):
     validation and test-retest reliability of a parent-administered
     questionnaire assessing nutrition risk of preschoolers. *Eur
     J Clin Nutr.* 2008;62:770-780.

36. Randall Simpson J, Gumbley J, Whyte K, et al. Development, reliability, and validity testing of Toddler NutriSTEP: a nutrition risk screening questionnaire for children 18-25 months of age. *Appl Physiol Nutr Metab.* 2015;40:977-886.

37. Rub G, Marderfeld L, Poraz I, et al. Validation of a nutritional screening tool for ambulatory use in pediatrics. *J Pediatr Gastroenterol Nutr.* 2016;62:771-775.

38. Food and Nutrition Service, United States Department of Agriculture. WIC Eligibility Requirements. Published May 11, 2018. www.fns.usda.gov/wic/wic-eligibility-requirements. Accessed August 13, 2018.

CHAPTER 3

Anthropometric Measurements

The most important parameter for evaluating the nutritional status of an infant, child, or adolescent is growth. Growth is reflected in a series of anthropometric indicators, including weight, length or height, head circumference (for infants and children less than 2 years old), and mid–upper arm circumference (MUAC). Other measurements, such as skinfold thickness, can help evaluate fat and muscle mass. Each measurement must be carefully taken using appropriate equipment, accurately recorded, and compared with either standards or reference data for age and growth trends for that particular patient/client.

For many years, growth has been evaluated by comparing the child's anthropometric measurements to growth standards using percentiles. However, in 2013, a new paradigm for diagnosing undernutrition in children across multiple settings using z scores was introduced.[1] Originally developed by the American Society for Parenteral and Enteral Nutrition (ASPEN), this approach has since been endorsed by both the American Academy of Pediatrics (AAP) and the Academy of Nutrition and Dietetics.[2,3] Protocols have since been implemented to evaluate the efficacy of this approach, and discussion of the challenges is ongoing.[4,5] Use and interpretation of z scores for diagnosing malnutrition in children are discussed later in this chapter.

Growth Charts

Growth charts have historically been the tools most often used to evaluate anthropometric indicators. Each chart is designed to plot one or more anthropometric indicators, including weight, length or height, head circumference, weight-for-length, and body mass index (BMI). The charts are gender and age specific and allow comparison of the indicator to population percentiles or z scores.

Understanding Percentile Curves

Growth charts consist of a series of percentile curves that represent the distribution of measurements of the population evaluated. A percentile is used to indicate how the child's measurement compares to other children his or her age. For example, a weight measurement at the 75th percentile means the child's weight is heavier than or equal to that of 75% of the children who are the same age and gender (ie, 75% of the children of the same age and gender weigh the same as or less than this child and 25% weigh more).

During the first year after birth, each child typically establishes his or her own growth pattern, with weight and length developing along a fairly consistent growth percentile channel. It is not uncommon for either minor deviations or growth spurts to occur. A child's growth channel may gradually shift over time as well, until genetic potential is reached. However, when either weight or length deviates substantially and repeatedly from the child's established growth percentiles, further assessment is indicated. Expected growth velocities (rates of gain in weight or length/stature) are discussed in the following sections.

Centers for Disease Control and Prevention Recommendations for Selecting Growth Charts

In the United States, the most widely available growth charts originate from the World Health Organization (WHO) and Centers for Disease Control and Prevention (CDC):

- The 2006 WHO growth charts for infants and children aged 0 to 60 months are based exclusively on data from breastfed infants and designed to reflect optimal growth of healthy breastfed infants and children living under conditions likely to favor achievement of their full genetic potential. The WHO charts can be used to assess all children, regardless of ethnicity, country of origin, socio-economic status, and type of feeding.[6]

- The 2000 CDC growth charts are intended as a growth reference at a point in time and were constructed using a cross-sectional sample of healthy American children.[7] In 2010, the CDC adopted the use of the WHO growth charts to assess all American infants from birth to 24 months of age because the WHO charts for this age group were based exclusively on longitudinal data from breastfed infants, a population that represents the optimal growth pattern for infants.[8]

In sum, the CDC recommends that health care providers do the following:[7,8]

- Use the WHO growth charts to monitor growth of infants and children aged 0 to 2 years in the United States. When using the WHO growth charts, measurements that are more than 2 standard deviations (SDs) above or below the mean, or the 2.3rd and 97.7th percentiles (labeled as the 2nd and 98th percentiles on the growth charts), are recommended for identification of children whose growth might be indicative of adverse health conditions.

- Use the CDC growth charts to monitor growth of children aged 2 years and older in the United States. Traditionally, measurements outside the 5th and 95th percentiles are used to identify potential risk or growth issues.

Types of Growth Charts Available from Centers for Disease Control and Prevention

WHO and CDC growth charts, as well as instructions for plotting anthropometric indicators, are available from the CDC website (www.cdc.gov/growthcharts). The types of charts recommended for use in the United States are summarized in Table 3.1 (page 32).[6,7] It is important to select the appropriate growth chart, keeping in mind the child's age, gender, and whether a recumbent length or standing height was measured. The WHO growth charts for ages 0 to 24 months use recumbent length, whereas standing height should be measured beginning at children aged 2 years and older and plotted on the CDC 2- to 20-year-old growth charts.

TABLE 3.1	Centers for Disease Control and Prevention and World Health Organization Age-Specific Growth Charts[a,6,7]
Age	**Charts**
0–24 mo	Weight-for-age
	Length-for-age
	Weight-for-length
	Head circumference-for-age
2–5 y	Weight-for-stature (optional; used in some public health settings)
2–20 y	Weight-for-age
	Stature-for-age
	Body mass index–for-age

[a]All charts are also gender specific. The Centers for Disease Control and Prevention (CDC) recommends use of World Health Organization charts for children aged 0 to 24 months and use of CDC charts for children older aged 2 years and older.

The CDC growth charts for children aged 2 to 20 years are available in English, Spanish, and French; some have two charts per page, with the grids scaled to metric units (centimeters and kilograms). The charts are available in sets, showing either the 5th to 95th percentile curves (intended for routine use in public health or clinical settings) or the 3rd to 97th percentile curves (for use by pediatric endocrinologists or to more closely monitor those growing at the outer percentiles). Individual charts are formatted with one chart per page, with the grids scaled to English units (inches and pounds).

Anthropometric Measurements

Growth Chart Software and Data Available from Centers for Disease Control and Prevention

The nutrition anthropometry software program NutStat from the CDC, contained within the program Epi Info, calculates percentiles and z scores for each measurement using the CDC reference data.[9] It is available to download at no charge from the CDC website.[9] Computer code to generate a database of anthropometric indices to use in Statistical Analysis System (SAS) software is also available to download from the CDC website.[9]

Specialized and Disease-Specific Growth Charts

Because prematurity, low birth weight, some medical conditions, and certain genetic syndromes can impact growth, specialized and disease-specific growth charts have been constructed to help track growth.

Growth Charts for Low-Birth-Weight and Premature Infants

The WHO growth charts are appropriate for term infants weighing more than 1,500 g at birth. For infants born prematurely (before 38 weeks of gestation), growth charts representing intrauterine growth rates should be used to assess postnatal growth.

- The Fenton growth charts were constructed using a meta-analysis of previously published international data and may be used to assess infants as young as 22 weeks of gestation.[10,11]

- The Olsen growth curves were constructed using data from infants born between 22 and 42 weeks of gestation in the United States and may best represent the current preterm infant population.[12]
- Lack of consensus, internationally, has resulted in continued efforts to develop growth standards for the premature infant population.[13,14] The International Fetal and Newborn Growth Consortium for the 21st Century (INTERGROWTH-21st) is a group of 27 institutions in 18 countries around the world working to develop universal perinatal growth standards. Information on their work is available at the INTERGROWTH-21st website (https://inter growth21.tghn.org).

Growth Charts for Children with Special Health Care Needs

Growth charts developed using appropriate populations are available for the following:

- achondroplasia[15-17]
- cerebral palsy[18-20]
- Cornelia de Lange syndrome[21]
- disproportionate growth disorders[22]
- Down syndrome[23]
- Ellis-van Creveld syndrome[24]
- Marfan syndrome[25,26]
- Morquio A disease[27]

- Noonan syndrome[28-30]
- Prader-Willi syndrome[31-34]
- Rett syndrome[35]
- Rubinstein-Taybi syndrome[36]
- Turner syndrome[37-39]
- Williams syndrome[40,41]
- Wolf-Hirschhorn syndrome[42]

When using disease-specific charts, it is important to consider the population and sample size on which they are based; many were developed using relatively small, cross-sectional populations of children varying in nutritional status. Some do not include growth curves for all the standard anthropometric indicators. These charts should be viewed as reference data rather than growth standards. CDC or WHO growth charts may be plotted along with the appropriate disease-specific chart.

Plotting and Interpreting a Child's Measurement on Growth Charts

Manual Plotting

To manually plot the recorded measurement(s) on the growth chart, perform the following:

1. On the horizontal (*x*) axis, find the child's age (or length, if plotting the weight-for-length chart). Using a straight edge, draw a vertical line from that point up to the growth curve.

2. On the vertical (y) axis, find the measured value (weight, length, height, head circumference, or BMI). Using a straight edge, draw a horizontal line across until it intersects the vertical line drawn.

3. Make a small dot at the intersection of the lines.

When plotted on the appropriate growth chart, the anthropometric measurement is typically described by the percentile line it is closest to or by the two lines it falls between. For example, a child's weight may be described as at the 50th percentile or as falling between the 25th and 50th percentiles.

Electronic Plotting

Growth charts were traditionally plotted manually. However, many facilities now use electronic medical records in which percentiles are calculated and growth charts are plotted electronically.[43,44] These applications offer the advantage of calculating an exact percentile or z score (eg, 15.9% or -1 z score) rather than a visual assessment made from a manually plotted chart (eg, 25th to 50th percentiles). The calculation of an exact percentile may eliminate plotting mistakes and facilitate the ability to identify deviations in growth more readily. However, minor deviations in growth may not be clinically significant and should be interpreted with caution.

Interpretation

Each individual typically grows along a given percentile channel over time; the growth of small-for-age children follows the lower percentile curves, whereas that of large-for-age children follows the upper percentile curves. Growth charts are also useful for evaluating and describing the velocity of changes in weight or length/ stature and head circumference (0 to 24 months). When growth either accelerates or decelerates such that the child's growth curve crosses percentiles, or when there is a significant discrepancy in percentiles for weight and height, the measurements should be repeated to verify their accuracy. If the measurements are found to be accurate, further investigation may be warranted.

z Scores

The z score is a statistical tool used to quantify how many standard deviations (SDs) away from the population mean a value lies. The population mean is analogous to the 50th percentile. Negative z scores reflect values below the mean, while positive z scores reflect values above the mean. Using z scores to describe anthropometric indicators is helpful because it allows an exact description of how far away from the mean the measurement lies. It may also be especially helpful in quantifying and tracking indicators that are below the 5th or above the 95th percentiles. The basic equation to calculate the z score is:

$$z \text{ Score} = \frac{x - \mu}{\sigma} = \frac{\text{measured value} - \text{population mean}}{\text{standard deviation of the mean}}$$

See Box 3.1 (pages 38 and 39) for resources for determining z scores of common anthropometric indicators used in assessing children.

Anthropometric
Measurements

BOX 3.1   Resources for Determining Anthropometric z Scores[3]

	Centers for Disease Control and Prevention Growth Charts	World Health Organization Growth Charts
STAT GrowthCharts: https://itunes.apple.com /ca/app/stat-growthcharts/id303475507 ?mt=8 (compatible with Apple Inc iPod Touch, iPhone, and iPad)	X	X
PediTools Home: www.peditools.org	X	
Epi Info NutStat: www.cdc.gov/growth charts/computer_programs.htm (available for download)	X	X

		X
Centers for Disease Control and Prevention website z score data files: www.cdc.gov /growthcharts/zscore.htm	X	
World Health Organization z score charts: www.who.int/childgrowth/standards/chart _catalogue/en/index.htm		X
World Health Organization Multicentre Growth Study website: www.who.int/childgrowth /software/en/		X

Age

Verifying or calculating an accurate age for the child is critical to the correct interpretation of anthropometric measurements and for plotting growth charts, especially for infants and toddlers. Many errors in interpretation of anthropometric indicators occur because the child's age is not calculated correctly.

Full-Term Infants and Children

Age should be determined to the nearest month for infants and to the nearest quarter-year for children aged 2 to 20 years. Detailed instructions for calculating the child's exact age and for rounding ages are provided in the CDC web module on the use of growth charts.[45]

Premature Infants and Young Children

To ensure a fair and appropriate comparison to norms for age, the age of infants and young children born prematurely should be corrected for the degree of prematurity. To correct for prematurity, do the following:

1. Subtract the infant's gestational age at birth from 40 weeks (term).
   Example: 40 weeks – 33 weeks' gestation = 7 weeks premature

2. Subtract the adjustment for prematurity
from the child's current chronological age.
Example: 18 months 2 weeks – 7 weeks
premature = 16 months 3 weeks corrected age

The child's measurements should then be compared to appropriate norms for the child's corrected age. Accelerated growth to achieve norms for chronological age, known as catch-up growth, occurs at different rates for each anthropometric indicator. From a practical standpoint, correction for prematurity may be used while the child is being plotted on the 0- to 24-month growth charts. It is important to note on the chart or assessment summary that corrected age was used or when the clinician stopped correcting for prematurity.

Head Circumference

Head circumference, also known as occipital frontal circumference (OFC), should be measured in infants and toddlers up to 24 to 36 months to the nearest 1 mm (0.1 cm) or ⅛ in. When evaluating the head circumference of a premature infant, correction for prematurity should be done until 18 months of age (see the preceding section Age in this chapter for instructions on how to correct for prematurity).

There is little relationship between head circumference and nutrition after 3 years. However, head circumference may continue to be measured in children with neurological impairment, particularly those at risk for hydrocephalus.

Available Growth Curves

Growth charts for evaluating OFC were published in 2006 by the WHO[46] for children aged 0 to 60 months. The CDC recommends use of the WHO growth curves for plotting head circumference in children younger than 24 months. A set of OFC reference curves that allows continuous monitoring of head circumference from birth to adulthood is also available.[47]

Measurement

To measure head circumference, use a flexible, non-stretchable ¼- to ½-in-wide plasticized measuring tape or an insertion tape.[48,49] The tape should encircle the head, crossing the forehead just above the eyebrows, continuing above the ears, and crossing the back of the head at its widest point. The goal is to find the largest circumference of the head.[49] Pull the tape to compress the hair. Any braids, barrettes, or hair ties that interfere with the measurement should be removed.[49]

For infants and children aged 0 to 24 months, the measured head circumference should be plotted on the WHO chart.

Evaluation

Brain Growth and Nutritional Status

Head circumference is an indicator of brain growth and may be affected by chronic undernutrition. Because brain growth is spared during periods of extended malnutrition, head circumference is the last of the three major measurements (following weight and length) to be affected by poor nutrition.[49]

Genetics

Head size is affected by familial genetics. Measuring the parents' heads and comparing them to adult head circumference references may be helpful in interpreting a child's head size, especially if it falls outside expected parameters.[50]

Microcephaly

Small head size (microcephaly) is usually defined as more than 2 standard deviations (SDs) below the mean. This value corresponds to the 3rd percentile on the WHO chart and the 2.3 percentile on the CDC chart. Note that in clinical practice, head circumference-for-age less than the 5th percentile on the CDC head circumference-for-age growth chart may be used to define microcephaly.[50] It may be caused by familial or other genetic factors or by prenatal or postnatal causes, including malnutrition. Poor head growth in the neonatal period of infants born less than 29 weeks of gestational age has been associated with significant neurodevelopmental delays.[51]

Macrocephaly

Large head size (macrocephaly) is similarly defined as more than 2 SDs above the mean or in clinical practice as greater than the 95th percentile on the head circumference-for-age growth chart.[52] Macrocephaly may also be caused by familial or genetic factors or by neurological pathology. It is not directly impacted by nutritional status.

Weight

Measurement

Weight should be measured using a calibrated beam-balance or electronic scale that can be easily zeroed and periodically calibrated. Weight may be measured in either pounds and ounces or kilograms and grams. Spring balance scales, such as bathroom scales, are not appropriate for obtaining weights for use in nutrition assessment.[48,49]

Infants

Scales to weigh infants should be capable of weighing in 0.01 kg (10 g) or in ½-oz increments. Infants and toddlers up to 18 months should be measured naked or wearing only a clean, dry diaper.[48,49]

Children Older Than 18 Months

Scales to weigh older children and adolescents should be capable of weighing in 0.1 kg (100 g) or in ¼-lb increments. Toddlers up to 24 months may continue to be weighed on infant scales as long as their weight does not exceed the maximum capacity of the scale. After 18 months, children should be measured wearing minimal clothing (underclothes, gown, or lightweight outer clothing) and no shoes. For serial measurements, whenever possible, the child should be weighed at the same time of day, in the same way, and on the same scale.[48,49]

Special Circumstances

Make note of any medical devices or equipment that cannot be removed, such as a brace, wheelchair, or pump. If possible, the equipment should be weighed separately and subtracted from the measured weight of the child with equipment.[48,49]

If the child is unable or is too active to sit or stand alone on the scale, the scale may be zeroed with the caregiver standing on it, and then the child's weight is measured while being held by the caregiver. Alternatively, a weight may be calculated by subtracting the caregiver's measured weight from the combined measured weight of the caregiver holding the child.[48,49]

Evaluation

Weight is an indicator of recent health and nutritional status. It is the first anthropometric measurement to reflect disruptions of either.[52]

Weight-for-Age

Weight-for-age, plotted on the appropriate WHO or CDC growth chart, is an indicator of an individual's weight compared with others of the same age and gender. It is most useful for tracking weight gain in infants and for helping to explain changes in weight-for-length/stature or BMI-for-age.[52]

Weight-for-age should *not* be used to classify a child as underweight or overweight. This can only be done using the weight-for-length/stature or BMI-for-age charts.[52] However, further evaluation should be considered for any child whose weight-for-age plots are below the 5th percentile or above the 95th percentile.

Velocity of Weight Gain

Weight gain in children is often described in terms of velocity of weight gain (the amount of weight the child has gained over a given period of time). Mean rates of weight gain are clinically useful to evaluate small weight gains of individuals between visits, which may be difficult to track on the growth chart over short intervals. Incremental weight gains based on WHO standards rather than CDC reference data have been demonstrated to be more appropriate for use in children from birth to 24 months of age.[53] Tables 3.2 through 3.5 (pages 47 to 50) provide weight gain velocities based on the WHO and CDC growth charts from birth to 20 years of age.[54,55]

TABLE 3.2 Mean Rates of Weight Gain for Boys Aged 0 to 24 Months[a],[54]

Age, mo	Mean Rate of Weight Gain	
	g/d	g/mo
0–3	33	996
3–6	17	527
6–9	10.5	321
9–12	8	246
12–15	7	214
15–18	6.6	201
18–21	6.4	195
21–24	6.1	185

[a]Based on weight gain at the 50th percentile of the World Health Organization growth charts

TABLE 3.3 Mean Rates of Weight Gain for Boys Aged 2 to 20 Years[a],[55]

Age, y	Mean Rate of Weight Gain	
	g/mo	kg/y
2–3	138[b]	1.6
3–4	150[c]	1.9
4–5	175	2.1
5–6	192	2.3
6–7	200	2.4
7–8	217	2.6
8–9	242	2.9

Continued on next page

TABLE 3.3	Mean Rates of Weight Gain for Boys Aged 2 to 20 Years[a,55] (cont.)	
Age, y	**Mean Rate of Weight Gain**	
	g/mo	kg/y
9–10	283	3.4
10–11	325	3.9
11–12	383	4.6
12–13	425	5.1
13–14	458	5.5
14–15	433	5.2
15–16	392	4.7
16–17	300	3.6
17–18	217	2.6
18–19	167	2.0
19–20	125	1.5

[a]Based on weight gain at the 50th percentile of the Centers for Disease Control and Prevention growth charts
[b]4.6 g/d
[c]5 g/d

TABLE 3.4	Mean Rates of Weight Gain for Girls Aged 0 to 24 Months[a,54]	
Age, mo	**Mean Rate of Weight Gain**	
	g/d	g/mo
0–3	28.5	868
3–6	16.0	493
6–9	10.0	308
9–12	7.5	235

TABLE 3.4   Mean Rates of Weight Gain for Girls Aged 0 to 24 Months[a,54] (cont.)

Age, mo	Mean Rate of Weight Gain	
	g/d	g/mo
12–15	7.0	214
15–18	7.0	210
18–21	6.5	203
21–24	6.0	190

[a]Based on weight gain at the 50th percentile of the World Health Organization growth charts

TABLE 3.5   Mean Rates of Weight Gain for Girls Aged 2 to 20 Years[a,55]

Age, y	Mean Rate of Weight Gain	
	g/mo	kg/y
2–3	150[b]	1.8
3–4	150[b]	1.9
4–5	183	2.2
5–6	192	2.3
6–7	208	2.5
7–8	242	2.9
8–9	275	3.3
9–10	325	3.9
10–11	367	4.4
11–12	367	4.4
12–13	350	4.2

Continued on next page

TABLE 3.5	Mean Rates of Weight Gain for Girls Aged 2 to 20 Years[a,55] (cont.)	
Age, y	Mean Rate of Weight Gain	
	g/mo	kg/y
13–14	292	3.5
14–15	225	2.7
15–16	150	1.8
16–17	108	1.3
17–18	83	1.0
18–19	100	1.2
19–20	75	0.9

[a]Based on weight gain at the 50th percentile of the Centers for Disease Control and Prevention growth charts
[b]5 g/d

For children in whom the goal is catch-up growth, weight gain should exceed the mean rate for age. However, the value of using weight or growth velocity as a predictor of child mortality in undernourished populations is controversial.[56,57] Conversely, research indicates that rapid weight gain between birth and 24 months of age may be associated with a higher risk for overweight and obesity later in childhood and adulthood.[58,59] Therefore, careful monitoring of weight gain as it relates to length or height is imperative.

Percentage of the Norm for Expected Weight Gain (<2 Years)

Since children up to 2 years of age are expected to be gaining weight continually, comparison of a child's actual weight gain over time to his or her expected weight gain over that same time interval may indicate malnutrition. Percentage of the norm for expected weight gain can be calculated using the following equation:

Percentage of the norm for expected weight gain

$$= \frac{(\text{expected weight gain} - \text{actual weight gain})}{\text{expected weight gain}} \times 100$$

The following percentage of the norm for expected weight gain in children less than 2 years are considered to be indicative of malnutrition:[3]

- Less than 75% of the norm for expected weight gain indicates mild malnutrition.
- Less than 50% of the norm for expected weight gain indicates moderate malnutrition.
- Less than 25% of the norm for expected weight gain indicates severe malnutrition.

Percentage Weight Loss (2 to 20 Years)

Any unintentional weight loss in children should be carefully evaluated. Percentage weight loss can be calculated using the following equation:

Percentage weight loss

$$= \frac{(\text{usual body weight} - \text{current body weight})}{\text{usual body weight}} \times 100$$

The following weight loss in children are considered to be indicative of malnutrition:[3]

- Loss of 5% of usual body weight indicates mild malnutrition.
- Loss of 7.5% of usual body weight indicates moderate malnutrition.
- Loss of 10% of usual body weight indicates severe malnutrition.

Weight-Age Equivalents

A weight-age equivalent is the age at which the child's current measured weight falls at the 50th percentile on the weight-for-age chart. It can be clinically useful to calculate this equivalent for children who gain weight at less than the expected rate for age as well as some children with special health care needs.[60]

For example, a 5-year-old child with poor weight gain may have a measured weight at the 50th percentile for a 3-year-old child. Clinically, it may be more appropriate to think of this child in terms of the expected growth rates of a 3-year-old rather than of a 5-year-old. This child may be described as being 5 years chronologically but as having the average weight of a 3-year-old.

Recumbent Length/Stature

Measurement of Recumbent Length

Recumbent length may be measured to the nearest 1 mm (0.1 cm) or ⅛ in, using a length board (infantometer) with an immovable perpendicular headboard and a movable perpendicular footboard. The measurement is taken from the top of the infant's head to the base of the heel (without shoes) while the infant is lying flat on his or her back, legs straight without bent knees, chin and toes pointing to the ceiling, with the head gently held in position.[48,49]

Recumbent length is typically measured for infants and toddlers up to age 24 months. The CDC recommends use of the WHO growth chart for plotting recumbent length in this age group.

Measurement of Standing Height/Stature

Stadiometer Method

Beginning at about age 24 months, standing height or stature may be measured to the nearest 1 mm (0.1 cm) or ⅛ in using a wall-mounted stadiometer (a vertical board with an attached rule and a movable horizontal headpiece fixed at a right angle to the vertical board). The stadiometer should be positioned over an uncarpeted floor. The height-measuring "stick" on a standing scale should never be used to measure stature because it is inaccurate and may injure the child.[48,49]

Height is measured with the child standing with heels, buttocks, shoulders, and back of the head touching the wall or stadiometer. The child should not be wearing shoes, the child's arms should be down at his or her sides, shoulders should be relaxed, and the child should look straight ahead.[48,49]

Methods for Estimating Stature

When older children are unable to stand or have contractures, other measurements can be made to estimate stature. These measurements include the following:

- crown-to-rump length
- sitting height
- arm span
- upper-arm or lower-leg length (knee height or tibial length)
- ulnar length

Any alternative methods of measurement should be noted in the child's health care record and on the corresponding growth chart.

Information on alternative measurement techniques, plotting, and the appropriate interpretation of these measurements has been developed by the University of Washington and the Maternal and Child Health Bureau.[61]

Evaluation

Length or stature is an indicator of a child's linear growth relative to age and is used to define shortness or tallness.[52] It is widely recognized as a marker of the overall well-being of a child, or a population of children.[62] The influence of genetics should be taken into consideration when evaluating a child whose stature is below or above the population norms.

Length-for-Age/Stature-for-Age

Length-for-age or stature-for-age, plotted on the appropriate WHO or CDC growth chart, is an indicator of the individual's height compared to others of the same age and gender.[52] It is important that the correct growth chart be used to interpret length or height:

- The 0-to-24-month WHO chart is used to plot recumbent length.
- The 2-to-20-year CDC chart is used to plot standing height.

Serial Measurements

Serial measurements over time can be used to track a child's linear growth. Mean rates of stature gain are clinically useful to evaluate the linear growth of an individual between visits, which may be difficult to track on the growth chart over short intervals. Similar to incremental weight gain, incremental increases in length based on WHO standards rather than CDC reference data have been demonstrated to be more appropriate for use in children from birth to 24 months of age.[53] Tables 3.6 to 3.9 (pages 56 to 59) provide linear gain velocities based on the WHO and CDC growth charts from birth to 20 years.[54,55]

TABLE 3.6	Mean Rates of Stature Gain for Boys Aged 0 to 24 Months[a,54]	
Age, mo	**Mean Rate of Stature Gain**	
	cm/d	cm/mo
0–3	0.120	3.80
3–6	0.068	2.10
6–9	0.048	1.50
9–12	0.042	1.25
12–15	0.037	1.13
15–18	0.034	1.03
18–21	0.032	0.97
21–24	0.280	0.87

[a]Based on increases in stature at the 50th percentile of the World Health Organization growth charts

TABLE 3.7	Mean Rates of Stature Gain for Boys Aged 2 to 18 Years[a,55]	
Age, y	**Mean Rate of Stature Gain**	
	cm/mo	cm/y
2–3	0.71	8.5
3–4	0.60	7.2
4–5	0.56	6.7

TABLE 3.7 Mean Rates of Stature Gain for Boys Aged 2 to 18 Years[a,55] (cont.)

Age, y	Mean Rate of Stature Gain	
	cm/mo	cm/y
5–6	0.54	6.5
6–7	0.53	6.4
7–8	0.51	6.1
8–9	0.47	5.7
9–10	0.43	5.1
10–11	0.41	4.9
11–12	0.46	5.5
12–13	0.59	7.0
13–14	0.64	7.8
14–15	0.51	6.1
15–16	0.30	3.6
16–17	0.15	1.8
17–18	0.07	0.9

[a]Based on increases in stature at the 50th percentile of the Centers for Disease Control and Prevention growth charts

TABLE 3.8 Mean Rates of Stature Gain for Girls Aged 0 to 24 Months[a,54]

Age, mo	Mean Rate of Stature Gain	
	cm/d	cm/mo
0–3	0.116	3.5
3–6	0.065	2.0
6–9	0.048	1.5

Continued on next page

TABLE 3.8 Mean Rates of Stature Gain for Girls Aged 0 to 24 Months[a],[54] (cont.)

Age, mo	Mean Rate of Stature Gain	
	cm/d	cm/mo
9–12	0.043	1.30
12–15	0.038	1.17
15–18	0.035	1.07
18–21	0.032	0.97
21–24	0.030	0.90

[a]Based on increases in stature at the 50th percentile of the World Health Organization growth charts

TABLE 3.9 Mean Rates of Stature Gain for Girls Aged 2 to 18 Years[a],[55]

Age, y	Mean Rate of Stature Gain	
	cm/mo	cm/y
2–3	0.74	8.9
3–4	0.57	6.8
4–5	0.58	6.9
5–6	0.58	7.0
6–7	0.56	6.8
7–8	0.51	6.1
8–9	0.44	5.3
9–10	0.42	5.1
10–11	0.50	6.0
11–12	0.60	7.2

TABLE 3.9   Mean Rates of Stature Gain for Girls Aged 2 to 18 Years[a,55] (cont.)

Age, y	Mean Rate of Stature Gain	
	cm/mo	cm/y
12–13	0.50	6.0
13–14	0.27	3.2
14–15	0.12	1.5
15–16	0.06	0.7
16–17	0.03	0.4
17–18	0.02	0.2

[a]Based on increases in stature at the 50th percentile of the Centers for Disease Control and Prevention growth charts

Length/Stature and Nutritional Status

Length/stature reflects long-term nutritional status and is affected more slowly than weight when a child experiences either undernutrition or overnutrition.

- *Undernutrition* may cause poor linear growth or stunting, resulting in the child's height being less than his or her genetic potential.
- *Overnutrition* may result in early maturation and accelerated linear growth, resulting in the child being tall for age and leading to earlier achievement of adult height.

Catch-Up Growth

In children for whom the goal is catch-up growth, stature gain should exceed the average rate for age. However, gains in stature occur more slowly than weight gains and may require an extended period of nutritional rehabilitation to achieve.

Short Stature

Factors that may contribute to short stature in children who are below the 5th percentile in length/stature-for-age include the following:

- malnutrition
- prenatal factors
- genetic disorders
- parental stature
- endocrine disorders
- other medical conditions, such as kidney failure

Age- and gender-specific standards have been developed to separate the genetic contribution of parental stature from other causes for children of short stature, including endocrine disorders. With these standards, the child's actual height is adjusted with a factor derived from the mean of each parent's height.[63] This adjustment should be considered for any child whose measured length or stature falls below the 5th percentile. Refer to the work of Himes and colleagues[63] for information about the estimation method and the data tables required to interpret findings. Note that multiple online calculators are available to predict a child's height potential based on midparental heights. However, these calculators are typically based on equations published in the work of Tanner and colleagues,[64] and, as Himes and colleagues[63] note, the Tanner equations are of limited clinical value for evaluation of US children because the population on which they are based was limited to white British children aged 2 to 9 years.

Slow Growth/Stunting

Children between the ages of 3 years and the onset of puberty who grow less than 4.5 cm (1.75 in) per year should be evaluated for causes of slower growth.[65] Familial short stature has a genetic basis and should be distinguished from stunting of linear growth as a result of chronic undernutrition.

Height-Age Equivalent

A height-age equivalent is the age at which the child's current measured length or stature would be at the 50th percentile on the length/stature-for-age chart. For children experiencing poor linear growth or stunting, it is sometimes clinically useful to calculate this equivalent.[60]

For example, a 5-year-old child experiencing linear growth stunting may have a measured height that is at the 50th percentile for a 3-year-old. Clinically, it may be more appropriate to think of this child in terms of the expected growth rates of a 3-year-old rather than of a 5-year-old.

Weight-for-Length/Height

Weight-for-length/height is an indicator used to identify overweight, underweight, or weight within normal
limits for infants up to the age of 24 months.[52] At a single point in time, weight-for-length is more meaningful
in children 0 to 24 months than either weight-for-age
or length-for-age alone. This is because the appropri-
ateness of the measured body weight is dependent on
the child's total body size (length), in addition to gender and age.

Weight-for-length/height is recommended as an
indicator of malnutrition at a single point in time for
children of all ages. Weight-for-length/height z scores
may be used to define degree of malnutrition as follows:

- Weight-for-length/height z score –1 to –1.9 indicates
  mild malnutrition.

- Weight-for-length/height z score –2 to –2.9 indicates moderate malnutrition.

- Weight-for-length/height z score –3 or greater indicates severe malnutrition.

Similarly, the WHO recommends using weight-for-
length/height to identify children with severe acute
malnutrition in global settings.[66]

In the United States, BMI-for-age should be used for
assessment in children aged 2 years and older to define
overweight and obesity (see the Body Mass Index section later in this chapter).

Serial Measurements

For children who are either below the 5th percentile or above the 95th percentile on the weight-for-length growth curves, serial measurements are important to determine whether this plot reflects a pathologic change in growth velocity or a consistent pattern of growth over time. A child who plots consistently below the 5th percentile on the weight-for-length chart but is growing along an established growth channel is of less concern than one whose weight-for-length is falling further below the curve over time. The first growth pattern may reflect a thin body habitus, whereas the second pattern may reflect growth faltering. However, it has been shown that as many as 62% of infants between birth and 6 months and 20% to 27% of children between 6 and 24 months crossed two major percentiles.[67] As a result, health care providers should use clinical judgment when evaluating changes in growth velocity.[68]

Likewise, a child who is consistently above the 95th percentile on the weight-for-length chart but is growing along an established growth channel is of less concern than one whose weight-for-length is increasing further above the curve. BMI-for-age (see the next section) is one way in which this phenomenon can be evaluated in terms of adiposity and risk of overweight for children aged 2 years and older.

Body Mass Index

BMI is a screening tool that is used to identify individuals who may be overweight or underweight.[69] BMI is an *indirect* measure of body fatness that has been shown to be related to adult adiposity and health risks.[70,71] In children, interpretation of BMI is gender and age specific. BMI is calculated using the individual's measured height and weight and one of the following equations:

$$BMI = [\text{weight (kg)/standing height}^2 \text{ (cm}^2)] \times 10,000$$

$$BMI = [\text{weight (lb)/standing height}^2 \text{ (in}^2)] \times 703$$

For children and adolescents aged 2 to 20 years, BMI should be plotted on the appropriate CDC BMI-for-age growth chart and monitored over time. One advantage of these charts is that they allow continued tracking of an individual's nutritional status into adulthood, where use of the BMI as a reflection of adiposity has been long established.

Plotting BMI-for-age is a more reliable method for predicting adiposity and risk of overweight/obesity than a visual assessment of the child. However, it should be noted that children who are athletic or muscular may have a calculated BMI indicative of overweight even though they lack adiposity. Measuring skinfold thickness may help to evaluate muscle and fat mass in these children. Likewise, children with various diagnoses that correlate with low muscle mass may be reflected as underweight though they have appropriate adiposity. Table 3.10 provides the current terms used to define BMI-for-age at both the lower and higher ranges of the BMI-for-age growth chart.

TABLE 3.10	Interpretation of Body Mass Index-for-Age[3,69]
−3 or greater z score	Severe malnutrition
−2 to −2.9 z score	Moderate malnutrition
−1 to −1.9 z score	Mild malnutrition
85th to <95th percentile	Overweight
≥95th percentile	Obese

Mid–Upper Arm Circumference

Measurement of a child's MUAC may be used to evaluate body stores of fat and muscle in infants, children, and adolescents. MUAC is considered to be a primary indicator of malnutrition when only one data point is available.[3,66] MUAC has been shown to be a better indicator of risk of mortality from pediatric malnutrition than weight-for-height.[72,73] Recent studies have demonstrated it to be an overall indicator of poor growth[74] as well as a reliable predictor of mortality of malnourished children.[75,76]

The measurement may also be useful in evaluating a child who is above the 95th percentile or one who has altered body composition secondary to neurological disease or in tracking body composition during nutritional rehabilitation from malnutrition.

Measurement

MUAC should be taken by an individual who has been trained in appropriate technique. MUAC is measured on the back side of the arm over the triceps muscle at the midpoint between the shoulder bone (acromion process) and the elbow (olecranon process). The elbow should be bent to facilitate finding the midpoint but should be straightened when the measurement is taken.

Evaluation

MUAC should be evaluated to assess risk for malnutrition using the following criteria:[3]

- MUAC z score −1 to −1.9 indicates mild malnutrition.
- MUAC z score −2 to −2.9 indicates moderate malnutrition.
- MUAC z score −3 or greater indicates severe malnutrition.

In 2017, two sets of data were published to allow calculation of z scores for MUAC. The first set is based on data from the 1999 to 2012 National Health and Nutrition Examination Surveys (NHANES) and includes reference ranges for children aged 2 months to 18 years.[77] This data has been used by Peditools.org to develop an MUAC z score calculator, allowing clinicians to access online (www.peditools.org) and easily include MUAC in their clinical assessment.[78] The second set is based on data from the NHANES between 1963 and 1994 and includes reference ranges for children aged 1 to 20 years, and it requires manual calculation of z score.[79]

Skinfold Thickness

Skinfold thickness measurements reflect energy stores as fat and can be used to evaluate nutritional status and body composition. Because individual differences in technique can mask true changes, serial measurements should be taken by the same person whenever possible. Protocols for taking anthropometric measurements, including MUAC and triceps skinfold (TSF), are available from the CDC (wwwn.cdc.gov/nchs/data/nhanes/2015-2016/manuals/2016_Anthropometry_Procedures_Manual.pdf).[80]

Measurement

Skinfold thickness measurements should be taken by an individual who has been trained in appropriate technique. The most commonly used skinfold measurement is the TSF, on the backside of the arm over the triceps muscle at the midpoint between the shoulder bone (acromion process) and the elbow (olecranon process). The elbow may be bent to facilitate finding the midpoint but should be straightened when the measurement is taken. TSF is measured at the midpoint using a skinfold caliper, with the arm hanging naturally by the subject's side. Subscapular skinfold thickness is measured at the base of the scapula using a skinfold caliper.

Evaluation

Reference curves are available to evaluate TSF thicknesses for children aged 18 months to 20 years, based on the same population used to construct the current CDC growth charts (see Tables 3.11 through 3.22, pages 69 to 80).[81] References for subscapular skinfold thickness are also available.[81]

TABLE 3.11	Smoothed Percentiles for Triceps Skinfold-for-Age, Millimeters: Boys Aged 1.5 to 4.9 Years[81]							
Percentile	Age, y							
	1.5–1.99	2.0–2.49	2.5–2.99	3.0–3.49	3.5–3.99	4.0–4.49	4.5–4.99
3rd	6.20	6.11	5.94	5.77	5.62	5.45	5.28
5th	6.55	6.46	6.29	6.12	5.96	5.79	5.61
10th	7.14	7.05	6.87	6.70	6.54	6.36	6.18
25th	8.27	8.17	7.99	7.82	7.65	7.48	7.29
50th	9.75	9.66	9.48	9.31	9.15	8.99	8.82
75th	11.52	11.44	11.28	11.14	11.01	10.88	10.74
85th	12.62	12.55	12.41	12.29	12.18	12.08	11.97
90th	13.43	13.37	13.25	13.14	13.06	12.98	12.90
95th	14.74	14.69	14.60	14.54	14.50	14.47	14.44
97th	15.66	15.63	15.57	15.53	15.53	15.54	15.56

Anthropometric
Measurements

TABLE 3.12 Smoothed Percentiles for Triceps Skinfold-for-Age, Millimeters: Boys Aged 5 to 7.9 Years[81]

Percentile	Age, y 5.00–5.49	5.50–5.99	6.00–6.49	6.50–6.99	7.00–7.49	7.50–7.99
3rd	5.09	4.91	4.73	4.59	4.49	4.44
5th	5.42	5.23	5.06	4.91	4.81	4.77
10th	5.99	5.8	5.62	5.47	5.38	5.35
25th	7.10	6.90	6.73	6.59	6.52	6.52
50th	8.63	8.46	8.30	8.20	8.17	8.24
75th	10.59	10.45	10.35	10.32	10.39	10.57
85th	11.86	11.76	11.7	11.73	11.88	12.17
90th	12.82	12.76	12.75	12.83	13.06	13.43
95th	14.42	14.44	14.51	14.71	15.07	15.62
97th	15.60	15.67	15.82	16.11	16.59	17.29

TABLE 3.13	Smoothed Percentiles for Triceps Skinfold-for-Age, Millimeters: Boys Aged 8 to 10.9 Years[81]						
Percentile	Age, y 8.00-8.49	8.50-8.99	9.00-9.49	9.50-9.99	10.00-10.49	10.50-10.99
3rd	4.43	4.45	4.49	4.55	4.6	4.63
5th	4.77	4.8	4.86	4.92	4.98	5.02
10th	5.36	5.42	5.50	5.59	5.67	5.73
25th	6.58	6.69	6.83	6.98	7.12	7.22
50th	8.39	8.59	8.84	9.10	9.35	9.55
75th	10.87	11.25	11.68	12.14	12.59	12.97
85th	12.59	13.11	13.7	14.33	14.95	15.49
90th	13.96	14.61	15.34	16.12	16.88	17.57
95th	16.36	17.25	18.25	19.33	20.4	21.39
97th	18.20	19.30	20.54	21.87	23.21	24.46

TABLE 3.14	Smoothed Percentiles for Triceps Skinfold-for-Age, Millimeters: Boys Aged 11 to 13.9 Years[81]						
Percentile	Age, y						
	11.00–11.49	11.50–11.99	12.00–12.49	12.50–12.99	13.00–13.49	13.50–13.99
3rd	4.63	4.60	4.53	4.44	4.33	4.20
5th	5.03	5.00	4.94	4.84	4.72	4.58
10th	5.75	5.73	5.66	5.56	5.42	5.26
25th	7.28	7.28	7.22	7.10	6.94	6.75
50th	9.68	9.73	9.70	9.58	9.39	9.16
75th	13.26	13.42	13.45	13.36	13.17	12.89
85th	15.91	16.19	16.30	16.25	16.07	15.78
90th	18.12	18.51	18.70	18.70	18.54	18.25
95th	22.21	22.83	23.20	23.33	23.24	22.97
97th	25.54	26.38	26.93	27.19	27.18	26.96

TABLE 3.15	Smoothed Percentiles for Triceps Skinfold-for-Age, Millimeters: Boys Aged 14 to 16.9 Years[81]						
Percentile	**Age, y**						
	14.00–14.49	**14.50–14.99**	**15.00–15.49**	**15.50–15.99**	**16.00–16.49**	**16.50–16.99**
3rd	4.06	3.94	3.84	3.75	3.70	3.66
5th	4.43	4.30	4.19	4.10	4.04	4.00
10th	5.10	4.95	4.82	4.72	4.65	4.61
25th	6.55	6.37	6.21	6.08	5.99	5.94
50th	8.91	8.67	8.46	8.30	8.18	8.13
75th	12.59	12.28	12.01	11.8	11.65	11.58
85th	15.44	15.10	14.79	14.54	14.37	14.30
90th	17.89	17.52	17.19	16.92	16.73	16.66
95th	22.60	22.20	21.83	21.53	21.33	21.25
97th	26.60	26.19	25.80	25.48	25.27	25.20

TABLE 3.16   Smoothed Percentiles for Triceps Skinfold-for-Age, Millimeters: Boys Aged 17 to 19.9 Years[81]

Percentile	Age, y 17.00–17.49	17.50–17.99	18.00–18.49	18.50–18.99	19.00–19.49	19.50–19.99
3rd	3.65	3.67	3.72	3.80	3.88	3.97
5th	3.99	4.01	4.07	4.15	4.24	4.34
10th	4.60	4.63	4.69	4.79	4.90	5.02
25th	5.93	5.98	6.07	6.19	6.34	6.50
50th	8.12	8.19	8.32	8.50	8.71	8.93
75th	11.59	11.69	11.88	12.15	12.46	12.79
85th	14.32	14.45	14.69	15.03	15.42	15.82
90th	16.69	16.84	17.13	17.53	17.98	18.45
95th	21.30	21.50	21.88	22.38	22.95	23.55
97th	25.27	25.52	25.96	26.56	27.23	27.93

TABLE 3.17 Smoothed Percentiles for Triceps Skinfold-for-Age, Millimeters: Girls Aged 1.5 to 4.9 Years[81]

Percentile	Age, y							
	1.50–1.99	2.00–2.49	2.50–2.99	3.00–3.49	3.50–3.99	4.00–4.49	4.50–4.99
3rd	6.23	6.18	6.09	6.00	5.91	5.82	5.72
5th	6.61	6.56	6.48	6.39	6.30	6.21	6.12
10th	7.23	7.19	7.12	7.04	6.96	6.88	6.8
25th	8.40	8.38	8.33	8.28	8.22	8.17	8.11
50th	9.91	9.91	9.91	9.90	9.89	9.88	9.87
75th	11.69	11.72	11.78	11.84	11.9	11.96	12.02
85th	12.77	12.82	12.92	13.03	13.14	13.25	13.37
90th	13.55	13.62	13.76	13.9	14.05	14.21	14.37
95th	14.79	14.89	15.10	15.31	15.53	15.75	16.00
97th	15.67	15.78	16.03	16.29	16.56	16.85	17.16

Anthropometric
Measurements

TABLE 3.18 Smoothed Percentiles for Triceps Skinfold-for-Age, Millimeters: Girls Aged 5 to 7.9 Years[81]

Percentile	Age, y 5.00–5.49	5.50–5.99	6.00–6.49	6.50–6.99	7.00–7.49	7.50–7.99
3rd	5.62	5.53	5.45	5.40	5.39	5.41
5th	6.03	5.94	5.87	5.83	5.82	5.86
10th	6.72	6.64	6.58	6.55	6.57	6.63
25th	8.05	8.00	7.98	7.99	8.05	8.18
50th	9.86	9.87	9.90	9.98	10.13	10.35
75th	12.10	12.19	12.31	12.51	12.78	13.15
85th	13.50	13.66	13.86	14.13	14.5	14.98
90th	14.55	14.76	15.02	15.36	15.81	16.37
95th	16.27	16.57	16.93	17.39	17.97	18.69
97th	17.49	17.86	18.30	18.85	19.54	20.38

TABLE 3.19 Smoothed Percentiles for Triceps Skinfold-for-Age, Millimeters: Girls Aged 8 to 10.9 Years[81]

Percentile	Age, y						
	8.00–8.49	8.50–8.99	9.00–9.49	9.50–9.99	10.00–10.49	10.50–10.99
3rd	5.46	5.54	5.63	5.72	5.80	5.87
5th	5.93	6.03	6.13	6.24	6.34	6.43
10th	6.73	6.86	7.00	7.14	7.28	7.40
25th	8.34	8.55	8.77	8.99	9.19	9.38
50th	10.63	10.96	11.3	11.64	11.97	12.27
75th	13.60	14.1	14.64	15.16	15.65	16.12
85th	15.55	16.18	16.84	17.50	18.12	18.69
90th	17.03	17.77	18.54	19.30	20.02	20.68
95th	19.52	20.44	21.40	22.34	23.23	24.05
97th	21.34	22.41	23.51	24.59	25.61	26.55

Anthropometric
Measurements

TABLE 3.20 Smoothed Percentiles for Triceps Skinfold-for-Age, Millimeters: Girls Aged 11 to 13.9 Years[81]

Percentile	Age, y 11.00–11.49	11.50–11.99	12.00–12.49	12.50–12.99	13.00–13.49	13.50–13.99
3rd	5.94	6.01	6.09	6.19	6.31	6.45
5th	6.51	6.60	6.70	6.82	6.95	7.11
10th	7.52	7.64	7.76	7.91	8.08	8.28
25th	9.57	9.76	9.95	10.16	10.4	10.66
50th	12.56	12.85	13.14	13.45	13.78	14.14
75th	16.56	16.98	17.40	17.84	18.29	18.76
85th	19.24	19.76	20.26	20.78	21.30	21.85
90th	21.31	21.90	22.47	23.04	23.63	24.22
95th	24.82	25.53	26.22	26.89	27.56	28.23
97th	27.42	28.23	28.99	29.73	30.46	31.18

TABLE 3.21	Smoothed Percentiles for Triceps Skinfold-for-Age, Millimeters: Girls Aged 14 to 16.9 Years[81]						
Percentile	Age, y						
	14.00–14.49	14.50–14.99	15.00–15.49	15.50–15.99	16.00–16.49	16.50–16.99	
3rd	6.61	6.79	6.98	7.19	7.40	7.61	
5th	7.30	7.50	7.71	7.94	8.17	8.40	
10th	8.49	8.73	8.98	9.24	9.51	9.78	
25th	10.95	11.26	11.57	11.90	12.23	12.56	
50th	14.52	14.91	15.31	15.72	16.12	16.52	
75th	19.25	19.75	20.23	20.71	21.19	21.65	
85th	22.40	22.95	23.48	24.00	24.51	24.99	
90th	24.81	25.40	25.96	26.50	27.03	27.53	
95th	28.88	29.52	30.12	30.69	31.23	31.74	
97th	31.88	32.54	33.16	33.74	34.29	34.80	

TABLE 3.22   Smoothed Percentiles for Triceps Skinfold-for-Age, Millimeters: Girls Aged 17 to 19.9 Years[81]

Percentile	Age, y 17.00–17.49	17.50–17.99	18.00–18.49	18.50–18.99	19.00–19.49	19.50–19.99
3rd	7.82	8.03	8.24	8.44	8.64	8.84
5th	8.64	8.86	9.09	9.31	9.53	9.76
10th	10.04	10.30	10.56	10.81	11.06	11.32
25th	12.88	13.19	13.50	13.81	14.12	14.43
50th	16.91	17.28	17.65	18.01	18.37	18.73
75th	22.09	22.52	22.93	23.33	23.73	24.13
85th	25.46	25.90	26.32	26.73	27.14	27.55
90th	28.00	28.45	28.87	29.28	29.69	30.11
95th	32.22	32.66	33.07	33.48	33.87	34.27
97th	35.26	35.69	36.09	36.48	36.86	37.24

Defining Malnutrition in Pediatrics

World Health Organization and United Nations Children's Fund

The WHO and the United Nations Children's Fund (UNICEF) Nutrition Section recommend the use of WHO growth standards to identify severe acute malnutrition (SAM) in infants and children.[66] The following diagnostic criteria are recommended for in children aged 6 to 60 months:

- weight-for-height < −3 SDs below the mean (see Table 3.23, pages 81 to85),
- mid-arm circumference < 155 mm, or
- bilateral edema

TABLE 3.23	World Health Organization or United Nations Children's Fund Weight-for-Height Diagnostic Criteria for Severe Acute Malnutrition in Children Aged 6 to 60 Months[66]	
Length, cm	**Weight Indicating SAM,[a] kg**	
	Girls	Boys
45	<1.9	<1.9
46	<2.0	<2.0
47	<2.2	<2.1

Continued on next page

TABLE 3.23 World Health Organization or United Nations Children's Fund Weight-for-Height Diagnostic Criteria for Severe Acute Malnutrition in Children Aged 6 to 60 Months[66] (cont.)

| Length, cm | Weight Indicating SAM,[a] kg | |
	Girls	Boys
48	<2.3	<2.3
49	<2.4	<2.4
50	<2.6	<2.6
51	<2.8	<2.7
52	<2.9	<2.9
53	<3.1	<3.1
54	<3.3	<3.3
55	<3.5	<3.6
56	<3.7	<3.8
57	<3.9	<4.0
58	<4.1	<4.3
59	<4.3	<4.5
60	<4.5	<4.7
61	<4.7	<4.9
62	<4.9	<5.1
63	<5.1	<5.3
64	<5.3	<5.5
65	<5.5	<5.7
66	<5.6	<5.9
67	<5.8	<6.1

TABLE 3.23	World Health Organization or United Nations Children's Fund Weight-for-Height Diagnostic Criteria for Severe Acute Malnutrition in Children Aged 6 to 60 Months[66] (cont.)	
Length, cm	**Weight Indicating SAM,[a] kg**	
	Girls	**Boys**
68	<6.0	<6.3
69	<6.1	<6.5
70	<6.3	<6.6
71	<6.5	<6.8
72	<6.6	<7.0
73	<6.8	<7.2
74	<6.9	<7.3
75	<7.1	<7.5
76	<7.2	<7.6
77	<7.4	<7.8
78	<7.5	<7.9
79	<7.7	<8.1
80	<7.8	<8.2
81	<8.0	<8.4
82	<8.1	<8.5
83	<8.3	<8.7
84	<8.5	<8.9
85	<8.7	<9.1
86	<8.9	<9.3
87	<9.2	<9.6

Continued on next page

TABLE 3.23 **World Health Organization or United Nations Children's Fund Weight-for-Height Diagnostic Criteria for Severe Acute Malnutrition in Children Aged 6 to 60 Months[66](cont.)**

Length, cm	Weight Indicating SAM,[a] kg	
	Girls	Boys
88	<9.4	<9.8
89	<9.6	<10.0
90	<9.8	<10.2
91	<10.0	<10.4
92	<10.2	<10.6
93	<10.4	<10.8
94	<10.6	<11.0
95	<10.8	<11.1
96	<10.9	<11.3
97	<11.1	<11.5
98	<11.3	<11.7
99	<11.5	<11.9
100	<11.7	<12.1
101	<12.0	<12.3
102	<12.2	<12.5
103	<12.4	<12.8
104	<12.6	<13.0
105	<12.9	<13.2
106	<13.1	<13.4
107	<13.4	<13.7
108	<13.7	<13.9

TABLE 3.23	World Health Organization or United Nations Children's Fund Weight-for-Height Diagnostic Criteria for Severe Acute Malnutrition in Children Aged 6 to 60 Months[66] (cont.)

Length, cm	Weight Indicating SAM,[a] kg	
	Girls	Boys
109	<13.9	<14.1
110	<14.2	<14.4
111	<14.5	<14.6
112	<14.8	<14.9
113	<15.1	<15.2
114	<15.4	<15.4
115	<15.7	<15.7
116	<16.0	<16.0
117	<16.3	<16.2
118	<16.6	<16.5
119	<16.9	<16.8
120	<17.3	<17.1

[a]Severe Acute Malnutrition (SAM) is defined as weight-for-height <−3 standard deviations from median

Academy of Nutrition and Dietetics and American Society for Parenteral and Enteral Nutrition

The Academy of Nutrition and Dietetics and the American Society for Parenteral and Enteral Nutrition issued a consensus paper on identification of malnutrition (undernutrition) using the following indicators: weight-for-height/length z score, BMI-for-age z score, length/height-for-age z score, MUAC z score, weight gain velocity, weight loss, deceleration in weight-for-length z score, and inadequate nutrient inake.[3]

Evaluation

Criteria to identify mild, moderate, and severe malnutrition with only a *single data point* are identified in Table 3.24.[3] Criteria to identify mild, moderate, and severe malnutrition with *two or more data points* are identified in Table 3.25 (page 88).[3] These indicators are intended to be used across the continuum of care, from acute to ambulatory settings. The goal of this effort is to standardize methods and speed the identification of children with malnutrition, resulting in earlier intervention.

TABLE 3.24 Criteria to Identify Pediatric Malnutrition with a Single Data Point			
Primary Indicators (z Score)	Mild Malnutrition (z Score)	Moderate Malnutrition (z Score)	Severe Malnutrition (z Score)
Weight-for-height	−1 to −1.9	−2 to −2.9	At or below −3
Body mass index-for-age	−1 to −1.9	−2 to −2.9	At or below −3
Length/height-for-age	No data	No data	At or below −3
Mid–upper arm circumference	≥−1 to −1.9	≥−2 to −2.9e	At or below −3 z score

Reprinted with permission from Becker PJ, Nieman Carney L, Corkins MR, et al. Consensus Statement of the Academy of Nutrition and Dietetics/America Society for Parenteral and Enteral Nutrition: indicators recommended for identification and documentation of pediatric malnutrition (undernutrition). *J Acad Nutr Diet.* 2014;114:1988-2000.[3]

TABLE 3.25 Criteria to Identify Pediatric Malnutrition with Two or More Data Points

Primary Indicators	Mild Malnutrition	Moderate Malnutrition	Severe Malnutrition
Weight gain velocity (<2 y of age)	<75% of the norm for expected weight gain	<50% of the norm for expected weight gain	<25% of the norm for expected weight gain
Weight loss (2–20 y of age)	5% of usual body weight	7.5% of usual body weight	10% of usual body weight
Deceleration in weight-for-length z score	Decline of 1 z score	Decline of 2 z score	Decline of 3 z score
Inadequate nutrient intake	51%–75% estimated energy/protein needs	26%–50% estimated energy/protein needs	≤25% estimated energy/protein needs

Reprinted with permission from Becker PJ, Nieman Carney L, Corkins MR, et al. Consensus Statement of the Academy of Nutrition and Dietetics/America Society for Parenteral and Enteral Nutrition: indicators recommended for identification and documentation of pediatric malnutrition (undernutrition). *J Acad Nutr Diet.* 2014;114:1988-2000.[3]

References

1. Mehta NM, Corkins MR, Lyman B, et al; American Society for Parenteral and Enteral Nutrition Board of Directors. Defining pediatric malnutrition: a paradigm shift toward etiology-related definitions. *J Parenter Enteral Nutr.* 2013;37:460-481

2. Statement of endorsement: defining pediatric Malnutrition. *Pediatrics.* 2013;132:e283.

3. Becker PJ, Nieman Carney L, Corkins MR, et al. Consensus Statement of the Academy of Nutrition and Dietetics/America Society for Parenteral and Enteral Nutrition: indicators recommended for identification and documentation of pediatric malnutrition (undernutrition). *J Acad Nutr Diet.* 2014;114:1988-2000.

4. Beer SS, Juarez MD, Vega MW, Canada NL. Pediatric malnutrition: putting the new definition and standards into practice. *Nutr Clin Pract.* 2015;30:609-624.

5. Bouma S. Diagnosing pediatric malnutrition: paradigm shifts of etiology-related definitions and appraisal of the indicators. *Nutr Clin Pract.* 2017;32:52-67.

6. World Health Organization. *WHO Child Growth Standards: Methods and Development.* Geneva, Switzerland: World Health Organization; 2006. www.who.int/childgrowth/standards /technical_report/en. Accessed January 24, 2018.

7. Growth charts. Centers for Disease Control and Prevention website. www.cdc.gov/growthcharts. Accessed January 24, 2018.

8. Centers for Disease Control and Prevention. Use of World Health Organization and CDC Growth charts for children aged 0-59 months in the United States. *MMWR.* 2010;59(no. RR-9):1-15.

9.   Computer programs. Centers for Disease Control and Prevention website. www.cdc.gov/nccdphp/dnpao/growth charts/resources/sas.htm. Accessed January 24, 2018.

10. Fenton TR. A new growth chart for preterm babies: Babson and Benda: Bendel chart updated with recent data and a new format. *BMC Pediatr.* 2003;3:13-22.

11. Fenton TR, Kim JH. A systematic review and meta-analysis to revise the Fenton growth chart for preterm infants. *BMC Pediatr.* 2013;13:59.

12. Olsen IE, Groveman SA, Clark RH, Zemel BS. New intrauterine growth curves based on United States data. *Pediatrics.* 2010;125:e214-e224.

13. Giuliani F, Cheikh Ismail L, Bertino E, et al. Monitoring postnatal growth of preterm infants: present and future. *Am J Clin Nutr.* 2016;103(suppl):635S-647S.

14. Villar J, Giuliana F, Bhutta ZA, et al. Postnatal growth standards for preterm infants: the Preterm Postnatal Follow-up Study of the INTERGROWTH–21st Project. *Lancet.* 2015;3:e681-e691.

15. Horton WA, Rotter JI, Rimoin DL, Scott CI, Hall JG. Standard growth curves for achondroplasia. *J Pediatr.* 1978;93:435-438.

16. Hoover-Fong JE, McGready J, Schulze KJ, Barnes H, Scott CI. Weight for age charts for children with achondroplasia. *Am J Med Genet Part A.* 2007;143A:2227-2235.

17. Hoover-Fong J, McGready J, Schulze K, Yewande Alade A, Scott CI. A height-for-age growth reference for children with achondroplasia: expanded applications and comparison with original reference data. *Am J Med Genet.* 2017;173A:1226-1230.

18. Brooks J, Day S, Shavelle R, Strauss D. Low weight, morbidity, and mortality in children with cerebral palsy: new clinical growth charts. *Pediatrics.* 2011;128:e299-e307.

Anthropometric
Measurements

19. Oeffinger D, Conaway M, Stevenson R, Hall J, Shapiro R, Tylkowski C. Tibial length growth curves for ambulatory children and adolescents with cerebral palsy. *Devel Med Child Neurol.* 2010;52:e195-e201.

20. Wright CM, Reynolds L, Ingram E, Cole TJ, Brooks J. Validation of US cerebral palsy growth charts using a UK cohort. *Devel Med Child Neurol.* 2017;59:933-938.

21. Kline AD, Barr M, Jackson LG. Growth manifestations in the Brachmann-de Lange syndrome. *Am J Med Genet.* 1993;47:1042-1049.

22. Fredriks AM, van Buuren S, van Heel WJM, Dijkman-Neerincx RHM, Verloove-Venhorick SP, Wit JM. Nationwide age references for sitting height, leg length, and sitting height/height ratio, and their diagnostic value for disproportionate growth disorders. *Arch Dis Child.* 2005;90:807-812.

23. Zemel BS, Pipan M, Stallings VA, et al. Growth charts for children with Down Syndrome in the United States. *Pediatrics.* 2015;136:e1204-e1211.

24. Verbeek S, Eilers PH, Lawrence K, Hennekam RCM, Versteegh FGA. Growth charts for children with Ellis-van Creveld syndrome. *Eur J Pediatr.* 2011;170:207-211.

25. Emery AH, Rimorin DL, eds. *Principles and Practice of Medical Genetics.* New York, NY: Churchill Livingston; 1983.

26. Papadatas CJ, Bartsocas CS, eds. *Endocrine Genetics and Genetics of Growth.* New York, NY: Alan R. Liss, Inc; 1985.

27. Montano AM, Tomatsu S, Brusius A, Smith M, Orii T. Growth charts for patients affected with Morquio A disease. *Am J Med Genet Part A.* 2008;146A:1286-1295.

28. Witt DR, Keena BA, Hall JG, Allanson JE. Growth curves for height in Noonan syndrome. *Clin Genet.* 1986;30:150-153.

29. Malaquias AC, Brasil AS, Pereira AC. Growth standards of patients with Noonan and Noonan-like syndromes with mutations in the RAS/MAPK pathway. *Am J Med Genet Part A*. 2012:158A:2700-2706.

30. Isojima T, Sakazume S, Hasegawa T, et al. Growth references for Japanese individuals with Noonan syndrome. *Pediatr Res*. 2016:79:543-548.

31. Butler MG, Sturich J, Lee J, et al. Growth standards in infants with Prader-Willi syndrome. *Pediatrics*. 2011;127:687-695.

32. Lee J, Isojima T, Chang MS, et al. Disease-specific growth charts for Korean infants with Prader-Willi syndrome. *Am J Med Genet Part A*. 2015;167A:86-94.

33. Butler MG, Lee J, Manzardo AM, et al. Growth charts for non-growth hormone treated Prader-Willi syndrome. *Pediatrics*. 2014;135:e126-e135.

34. Butler MG, Lee J, Cox DM, et al. Growth charts for Prader-Willi syndrome during growth hormone treatment. *Clin Pediatr*. 2016;55:957-974.

35. Tarquinio DC, Motil KJ, Hou W, et al. Growth failure and outcome in Rett syndrome: specific growth references. *Neurology*. 2012;79:1653-1661.

36. Beets L, Rodriquez-Fonseca C, Hennekam RC. Growth charts for individuals with Rubenstein-Taybi syndrome. *Am J Med Genet Part A*. 2014;164A:2300-2309.

37. Lyon AJ, Preece MA, Grant DB. Growth curves for girls with Turner syndrome. *Arch Dis Child*. 1985;60:932-935.

38. Ranke MB, Pfluger H, Rosendahl W, et al. Turner syndrome: spontaneous growth in 150 cases and review of the literature. *Eur J Pediatr*. 1983;141:81-88.

39. Isojima T, Yokoya S. Development of disease-specific growth charts in Turner syndrome and Noonan Syndrome. *Ann Pediatr Endocrinol Metab*. 2017;22:240-246.

40. Morris CA, Demsey SA, Leonard CO, Dilts C, Blackburn BL. Natural history of Williams syndrome: physical characteristics. *J Pediatr.* 1988;113:318-326.

41. Martin NDT, Smith WR, Cole TJ, Preece MA. New height, weight and head circumference charts for British children with Williams syndrome. *Arch Dis Child.* 2007;92:598-601.

42. Antonius T, Draaisma J, Levtchenko E, Knoers N, Renier W, van Ravenswaaij C. Growth charts for Wolf-Hirschhorn syndrome (0-4 years of age). *Eur J Pediatr.* 2008;167:807-810.

43. Rosenbloom ST, Qi X, Riddle WR, et al. Implementing pediatric growth charts into an electronic health record system. *J Am Med Inform Assoc.* 2006;13:302-308.

44. Andrews ET, Wootton S, Cable D, Marchant A, Miller H, Davies JH. Embedding electronic growth charts into clinical practice at a children's hospital. *Arch Dis Child Educ Pract Ed.* 2018;103(2):82-84.

45. Use and interpretation of the CDC growth charts. Centers for Disease Control and Prevention website. www.cdc.gov/nccdphp/dnpa/growthcharts/resources/growthchart.pdf. Accessed August 13, 2018.

46. WHO Child Growth Standards Methods and Development: Head Circumference-for-Age, Arm Circumference-for-Age, Triceps Skinfold-for-Age and Subscapular Skinfold-for-Age. World Health Organization website. www.who.int/nutrition/publications/childgrowthstandards_technical_report_2/en. Accessed January 24, 2018.

47. Rollin JD, Collins JS, Holden KR. United States head circumference growth reference charts: birth to 21 years. *J Pediatr.* 2010;156:907-913.

48. Maternal and Child Health Bureau. Accurately weighing and measuring infants, children and adolescents: equipment. University of Washington website. http://depts.washington.edu/growth/index.htm. Accessed January 24, 2018.

49. Maternal and Child Health Bureau. Accurately weighing and measuring infants, children and adolescents: technique. University of Washington website. http://depts.washington.edu/growth. Accessed January 24, 2018.

50. Maternal and Child Health Bureau. Interpreting growth in head circumference. University of Washington website. http://depts.washington.edu/growth/ofc/text/intro.htm. Accessed January 24, 2018.

51. Raghuram K, Yang J, Church PT, et al. Head growth trajectory and neurodevelopmental outcomes in preterm neonates. *Pediatrics*. 2017;140(1):e20170216. doi:10.1542/peds.2017-0216.

52. Overview of the CDC growth charts. Centers for Disease Control and Prevention website. www.cdc.gov/nccdphp/dnpao/growthcharts. Accessed January 24, 2018.

53. de Onis M, Siyam A, Borghi E, Onyango AW, Piwoz E, Garza C. Comparison of the World Health Organization Growth Velocity Standards with existing US reference data. *Pediatrics*. 2011;128:e18-e26.

54. World Health Organization. *WHO Child Growth Standards: Methods and Development. Growth Velocity Based on Weight, Length, and Head Circumference*. Geneva, Switzerland: World Health Organization; 2009. www.who.int/nutrition/publications/childgrowthstandards_technical_report_3/en. Accessed January 24, 2018.

55. Percentile data files with LMS values. Centers for Disease Control and Prevention website. www.cdc.gov/growthcharts/percentile_data_files.htm. Accessed January 24, 2018.

56. Schwinger C, Fadnes LT, Van den Broeck J. Using growth velocity to predict child mortality. *Am J Clin Nutr*. 2016;103:801-807.

57. Schwinger C, Fadnes LT, Shrestha SK, et al. Predicting undernutrition at age 2 years with early attained weight and length compared with weight and length velocity. *J Pediatr.* 2017;182:127-132.

58. Chomtho S, Wells JCK, Williams JE, Davies PSW, Lucas A, Fewtrell MS. Infant growth and later body composition: evidence from the 4-component model. *Am J Clin Nutr.* 2008;87:1776-1784.

59. Gungor DE, Paul IM, Birch LL, Bartok CJ. Risky vs rapid growth in infancy. *Arch Pediatr Adolesc Med.* 2010;164:1091-1097.

60. Behavioral Health Nutrition Dietetic Practice Group and Pediatric Nutrition Practice Group. *Academy of Nutrition and Dietetics Pocket Guide to Children with Special Health Care and Nutritional Needs.* Chicago, IL: Academy of Nutrition and Dietetics; 2012.

61. Maternal and Child Health Bureau. The CDC growth charts for children with special health care needs. University of Washington website. http://depts.washington.edu/growth/cshcn/text/pagela.htm. Accessed January 24, 2018.

62. de Onis M, Branca F. Childhood stunting: a global perspective. *Matern Child Nutr.* 2016;12(suppl 1):12-26.

63. Himes JH, Roche AF, Thissen D, Moore WM. Parent-specific adjustments for evaluation of recumbent length and stature of children. *Pediatrics.* 1985;75:304-313.

64. Tanner JM, Goldstein H, Whitehouse RH. Standards for children's heights at ages 2-9 years allowing for height of parents. *Arch Dis Child.* 1970;45:755-762.

65. Duck SC. Identification and assessment of the slowly growing child. *Am Fam Physician.* 1996;53:2305-2312.

66. *WHO Child Growth Standards and the Identification of Severe Acute Malnutrition in Infants and Children.* Geneva, Switzerland: A Joint Statement by the World Health Organization and the United Nations Children's Fund; 2009. www.who.int/nutrition/publications /severemalnutrition/9789241598163_eng.pdf. Accessed January 24, 2018.

67. Mei Z, Grummer-Strawn LM, Thompson D, Dietz WH. Shifts in percentiles of growth during early childhood: analysis of longitudinal data from the California Child Health and Development Study. *Pediatrics.* 2004;113:e617-e627.

68. Jaffe AC. Failure to thrive: current clinical concepts. *Pediatr Rev.* 2011;32:100-107.

69. Using the CDC BMI-for-Age Growth Charts to Assess Growth in the United States among Children and Teens Aged 2 years to 20 years. Centers for Disease Control and Prevention website. www.cdc.gov/nccdphp/dnpao/growthcharts /training/bmiage/index.html. Accessed January 24, 2018.

70. Freedman DS, Kahn LK, Serdula MK, Dietz WH, Srinivasan SR, Berenson GS. The relation of childhood BMI to adult adiposity: the Bogalusa Heart Study. *Pediatrics.* 2005;115:22-27.

71. Freedman DS, Kahn LK, Dietz WH, Srinivasan SR, Berenson GS. Relationship of childhood obesity to coronary heart disease risk factors in adulthood: the Bogalusa Heart Study. *Pediatrics.* 2001;108:712-718.

72. Briend A, Marie B, Fontaine O, Garenne M. Mid-upper arm circumference and weight-for-height to identify high-risk malnourished under-five children. *Matern Child Nutr.* 2012;8:130-133.

73. Rasmussen J, Andreson A, Fisker AB, et al. Mid-upper-arm-circumference and mid-upper-arm circumference z-score: the best predictor of mortality? *Eur J Clin Nutr.* 2012;66:998-1003.

74. Grijalva-Eternod CS, Wells JCK, Girma T, et al. Midupper arm circumference and weight-for-length z scores have different associations with body composition: evidence from a cohort of Ethiopian infants. *Am J Clin Nutr.* 2015;102:593-599.

75. Sachdeva S, Dewan P, Shah D, Malhotra RK, Gupta P. Mid-upper arm circumference v. weight-for-height Z-score for predicting mortality in hospitalized children under 5 years of age. *Public Health Nutr.* 2016;19:2513-2520.

76. Mwangome M, Ngari M, Fegan G, et al. Diagnostic criteria for severe acute malnutrition among infants aged under 6 mo. *Am J Clin Nutr.* 2017;105:1415-1423.

77. Abel-Rahman SM, Bi C, Thaete K. Construction of lambda, mu, sigma values for determining mid-upper arm circumference z scores in U.S. children aged 2 months through 18 years. *Nutr Clin Pract.* 2017;32:68-76.

78. Peditools. http://peditools.org. Accessed January 25, 2018.

79. Addo OY, Himes JH, Zemel BS. Reference ranges for midupper arm circumference, upper arm muscle area, and upper arm fat area in US children and adolescents aged 1-20 y. *Am J Clin Nutr.* 2017;105:111-120.

80. *National Health and Nutrition Examination Survey Anthropometry Procedures Manual.* Washington, DC: Centers for Disease Control and Prevention; 2016. wwwn.cdc.gov/nchs/data/nhanes/2015-2016/manuals/2016_Anthropometry_Procedures_Manual.pdf. Accessed August 13, 2018.

CHAPTER 4

Client History

A complete history of factors affecting a child's nutritional status is essential to making the correct nutrition diagnosis and to developing an appropriate nutrition care plan. Information about medical/health history (including prenatal and birth history, if relevant, and medication and supplement use) helps identify physiologic and metabolic causes of compromised nutritional status. Evaluation of development, including the sexual maturation of teenagers, adds information that can alert the clinician of the need to adjust assessment parameters, such as expected feeding skills of an infant or toddler or the nutrient requirements of an adolescent. Assessment of the family environment puts the child's nutritional status into context and helps to pinpoint the etiology of potential nonphysiologic causes of nutrition abnormalities.

Medical/Health History

A complete medical/health history of the infant, child, or adolescent should be noted as part of the nutrition assessment. Components of a pediatric nutrition–oriented medical history are listed in Box 4.1.[1]

BOX 4.1 Components of a Pediatric Nutrition–Oriented Medical History[1]
Chief complaint
Current health status
Chronic disease status
Psychiatric history
Surgeries
Diagnostic procedures
Medical therapies
Family health history
Oral health history
Medications and supplements
Sexual maturity rating (Tanner stage) in adolescents

Growth history, including previous measures of height, weight, and head circumference, if appropriate, should be obtained, plotted on the corresponding growth charts, and evaluated for trends (see Chapter 3).

For infants and young children, it is important to take a history of any emesis (including spitting up) and stool patterns.

Prenatal and Birth History

For infants, any significant prenatal and birth history should be recorded. Maternal use of alcohol or drugs, prenatal exposure to viral illnesses, current diet if breastfeeding, and history of gestational diabetes and prenatal weight gain are all important factors to note.

Birth-related factors, such as birth weight and length, prematurity, medical treatments required at birth, length of hospitalization, adjustment to the home environment, initial feeding method, and formula choice (if infant is formula fed), should be noted.

Medications and Supplements

The medical/health history should include a review of all prescription and over-the-counter medications, vitamins, minerals, and herbal or other supplements taken by the child over the last several weeks or months. Many medications and supplements affect nutrient status, either by interacting with food consumed or by causing metabolic alterations that affect nutritional status (see Box 4.2).[2]

Client History

BOX 4.2   Drug-Nutrient Interactions

Antibiotics

Nutrients affected: Minerals, fats, proteins

Overall effect: Temporary decrease in absorption (resulting from diarrhea, nausea, and/or vomiting); destroys "good" intestinal bacteria flora.

Prevention: Acidophilus and other probiotics may counteract loss of intestinal flora.

Anticonvulsants

Nutrients affected: Vitamins D, K, B-6, and B-12; folate; calcium

Overall effect: Decrease in nutrient absorption or stores.

Prevention: Recommend diet high in these nutrients. Vitamin and mineral supplements may be appropriate; seek physician approval as supplementation may influence drug effectiveness.

Cardiac Medications (Diuretics)

Nutrients affected: Potassium, magnesium, calcium, folate

Continued on next page

BOX 4.2 Drug-Nutrient Interactions (cont.)

Cardiac Medications (Diuretics) (cont.)

Overall effect: Loss or depletion of nutrient stores;
                         some diuretics can produce these
                         effects; may also cause nausea,
                         diarrhea, and vomiting that lead to
                         reduced food intake.

Prevention: Recommend foods and fluids high in
                         potassium and magnesium. Suggest
                         strategies to help with decreased
                         appetite.

Corticosteroids

Used with asthma, arthritis, gastrointestinal disease, cardiac
disease, cancer, muscular dystrophy, and so on

Nutrients affected: Calcium, phosphorus, glucose, vita-
                         min D, protein, sodium, water, zinc,
                         vitamin C, potassium

Overall effect: Long-term use can cause stunting
                         of growth, can deplete calcium and
                         phosphorus that can result in bone
                         loss, and can affect glucose levels.
                         May also increase appetite, leading
                         to weight gain. Also can cause fluid
                         retention and require monitoring of
                         sodium. Can cause peptic disease,
                         vomiting/diarrhea.

Client History

| BOX 4.2 | **Drug-Nutrient Interactions (cont.)** |

Prevention: Monitor weight, laboratory values. Supplement with calcium and vitamin D.

Laxative/Bulk Agents

Nutrients affected: Fat-soluble vitamins

Overall effect: Some are bulking agents, and others are laxatives. Some laxatives may deplete fat-soluble vitamins when used long term.

Prevention: Encourage a diet high in fiber and fluid to wean child off medication. Regimen may need to be altered if a child changes the amount of fiber or fluid intake. Check with physician for alternative medication that will not deplete stores. Encourage weight-bearing exercise.

Anti–Gastroesophageal Reflux Disease Medications

Nutrients affected: Vitamin B-12, iron, calcium

Overall effect: Can cause long-term loss of iron, vitamin B-12, and calcium. May cause nausea and diarrhea.

Continued on next page

BOX 4.2   Drug-Nutrient Interactions (cont.)

Anti–Gastroesophageal Reflux Disease Medications (cont.)

Prevention: Recommend diet high in these nutri-
                         ents; monitor laboratory values.

Stimulants

Used for attention deficit hyperactivity disorder.

Overall effect: Can decrease appetite and cause
                         weight loss; may affect overall
                         growth.

Prevention: Have child eat before each medi-
                         cation dosage, if possible. Choose
                         meals at which they are most hun-
                         gry, and encourage larger amounts
                         of intake at those times. Monitor
                         growth, and discuss with physician if
                         it is affected.

Sulfonamides

Used in spina bifida.

Nutrients affected: Vitamin C, protein, folate, iron

Overall effect: Promotes crystallization of large
                         doses of vitamin C in the blad-
                         der, inhibits protein synthesis, and
                         decreases serum folate and iron.

Client History

BOX 4.2 Drug-Nutrient Interactions (cont.)

Prevention:	Avoid supplementation of vitamin C in large doses (>1,000 mg). Increase intake of high-folate foods. Practitioners are unable to use color or odor of urine as a determinant of hydration status.

Tranquilizers

Overall effect:	Increases appetite; results in excessive weight gain.
Prevention:	Recommend a low-calorie diet, if appropriate. Monitor weight.

Antipsychotics

Nutrients affected:	Sodium, potassium
Overall effect:	Decreases nutrient absorption. Increases weight gain.
Prevention:	Monitor weight and laboratory test values.

Reprinted with permission from Corkins KG, Wittenbrook W, eds. Behavioral Health Nutrition Dietetic Practice Group and Pediatric Nutrition Practice Group. *Academy of Nutrition and Dietetics Pocket Guide to Children with Special Health Care and Nutritional Needs.* 2nd ed. Chicago, IL: Academy of Nutrition and Dietetics; in press.[2]

As with adults, the use of complementary and alternative therapies in infants, children, and adolescents is on the rise.[3] Some parents use botanical treatments to treat minor illnesses. The use of alternative therapies, including botanical treatments, may be more common in some cultural groups. For example, chamomile is sometimes used to treat colic, especially among Hispanic parents.[3] Families may also use botanical treatments for more serious chronic illnesses and conditions, such as cancer and certain developmental disorders. All complementary and alternative therapies should be noted and explored for possible nutritional consequences.

Development

Chronological age is not always a reliable marker of expected growth or nutritional status. Delays in motor or cognitive development may affect nutrient intake or growth or may indicate a decline in functional status as a result of malnutrition, and they should be noted.

Motor Development

Table 4.1 outlines motor development milestones in the first 2 years of life, as identified by the World Health Organization.[4] (See Boxes 5.3 and 5.4 on pages 125 to 130 for the normal progression of physical skills related to eating.)

TABLE 4.1 Windows of Achievement for Six Gross Motor Development Milestones[4]

Milestone	Boundaries (Age in Months)
Sitting without support	3.8–9.2
Standing with assistance	4.8–11.4
Hands-and-knees crawling	5.2–13.5
Walking with assistance	6.0–13.7
Standing alone	6.9–16.9
Walking alone	8.2–17.6

Cognitive Development

For information about cognitive delays, ask the child's caregiver or check the medical record.

Sexual Development

For adolescents, sexual maturation is a useful way to assess the stage of puberty and corresponding nutrient needs. Development of secondary sex characteristics can be evaluated using sexual maturity rating, often called Tanner staging. Table 4.2 (page 108) provides a summary of the stages of pubertal development.[5]

TABLE 4.2   Sexual Maturity Rating[5]

Stage	Males	Females
1	Prepubertal	Prepubertal
2	Enlargement of scrotum and testes, scrotal skin reddens	Breast budding with areolar enlargement
	Sparse growth of slightly pigmented hair at base of penis	Sparse growth of slightly pigmented hair along labia
3	Further growth of the testes and scrotum, enlargement of the penis (increased length and width)	Further enlargement of breasts and areola
		Pubic hair is darker, coarser, curlier, and more dispersed
	Darker, coarser, curlier, more dispersed pubic hair	
4	Still further growth of genitalia	Projection of the areola and papilla to form a secondary mound
	Adult-type pubic hair, but not extending to thighs	Adult-type pubic hair, but not extending to thighs
		Menarche[a]
5	Adult genitalia	Adult breast with projection of papilla only
	Adult pubic hair, extending to thighs	Adult pubic hair, extending to thighs

[a] Females typically experience most linear growth before the onset of menarche. They grow on average only 2 inches after menarche. However, girls who enter puberty at an earlier age may experience more linear growth after menarche than those who are older at the start of puberty

Client History

Using the Tanner stages of pubertal development, energy and protein needs can be assessed based on developmental stage rather than chronological age alone. Females experience their most rapid growth in height (3 to 5 in) between stages 2 and 3 and have their highest energy requirement (2,300 to 3,000 kcal/day) during this interval.[5] Males experience their most rapid growth in height (6 to 8 in) between stages 3 and 4 and have their highest energy requirement (2,800 to 3,500 kcal/day, depending on activity) during this interval.[5]

Family and Community Environment

Most children do not make food- and nutrition-related choices independently. As a result, understanding the family, cultural, and social environment is an essential part of the nutrition assessment (see Box 4.3).[6,7]

BOX 4.3 Family-Related Social and Behavioral Factors Affecting Nutritional Status[6,7]

Members of the household (include information on multiple households where appropriate)

Caregivers for the child (include day care providers, after-school care providers, stepparents, and grandparents)

Continued on next page

BOX 4.3 Family-Related Social and Behavioral Factors Affecting Nutritional Status[6,7] (cont.)

Caregivers' ability to procure and prepare food

Setting for meals and snacks (eg, seated at the table, in front of the television, or at fast-food restaurants)

Mealtime environment (include whether family members eat as a group or alone)

Mealtime atmosphere (eg, pleasant conversation vs loud arguments)

Caregivers' approach to child's food preferences, ability to make choices, and regulate intake (eg, pressure to eat or restriction of foods)

Caregivers' expectations of the child's mealtime behavior

Financial resources, participation in food assistance programs, refrigeration and cooking facilities, transportation and access to food

Cultural or religious food preferences, dietary habits, or feeding practices

Family history of eating disorders or obesity (as appropriate to the assessment)

Family dysfunction (eg, alcohol or drug dependence)

Emotional distress or depression

Caregivers' attitudes toward and expectations for the child's health and nutritional status

Physical activity habits and media-viewing behaviors of the family

In addition, many specific health- and food-related behaviors have their origin in the cultural heritage of the client. Clinicians working with specific immigrant communities should familiarize themselves with the beliefs and customs of their client population and also gain an understanding of typical meal patterns and feeding rituals.[7]

References

1. Marian MJ. Client history. In: Charney P, Malone A, eds. *Academy of Nutrition and Dietetics Pocket Guide to Nutrition Assessment*. 3rd ed. Chicago, IL: Academy of Nutrition and Dietetics; 2015.

2. Corkins KG, Wittenbrook W, eds. Behavioral Health Nutrition Dietetic Practice Group, Pediatric Nutrition Practice Group. *Academy of Nutrition and Dietetics Pocket Guide to Children with Special Health Care and Nutritional Needs*. 2nd ed. Chicago, IL: Academy of Nutrition and Dietetics; in press.

3. Westerdahl J. Botanicals in pediatrics. In: Samour PQ, King K, eds. *Handbook of Pediatric Nutrition*. 4th ed. Sudbury, MA: Jones and Bartlett; 2012.

4. WHO Multicentre Growth Reference Study Group. WHO Motor Development Study: windows of achievement for six gross motor development milestones. *Acta Paediatr.* 2006;450(suppl):S86-S95.

5. Adolescent nutrition. In: Kleinman RE, Greer FR, eds. *Pediatric Nutrition Handbook*. 7th ed. Elk Grove Village, IL: American Academy of Pediatrics; 2014:175-187.

6.   Lucas B, Ogata B, Feucht S. Normal nutrition from infancy through adolescence. In: Samour PQ, King K, eds. *Handbook of Pediatric Nutrition*. 4th ed. Boston, MA: Jones and Bartlett; 2012:103-126.

7.   Cultural considerations in feeding infants and young children. In: Kleinman RE, Greer FR, eds. *Pediatric Nutrition Handbook*. 7th ed. Elk Grove Village, IL: American Academy of Pediatrics; 2014:219-240.

Client History

CHAPTER 5

Food and Nutrition History

Food and nutrition history plays a key role in pediatric nutrition assessment. The diet history is used to evaluate usual intake for the purpose of assessing nutritional adequacy, abnormal eating behaviors, and feeding difficulties. Because dietary intake and feeding skills change dramatically in the years from infancy through adolescence, it is critical that this part of the assessment takes into account the child's age, the normal progression of feeding skills for age, and typical eating patterns for age. Food intake patterns, along with appropriate portions for age, provide a basis for comparison of usual dietary intake with recommended intake.

Diet History

The reliable diet history of an infant, child, or adolescent provides a wealth of information critical to making an accurate nutrition diagnosis (see Box 5.1).[1,2] From the diet history, the clinician is able to assess macronutrient and micronutrient intakes, food consumption patterns, food preferences, and the feeding environment. The diet history may also help to explain clinical symptoms of nutrient intake abnormalities or may point to the need for laboratory assessment.

BOX 5.1   Key Elements of a Pediatric Diet History

Type, brand name, and amount of food, beverages, or formula actually consumed at a meal or snack

Preparation methods for foods and formula (including type of water used, eg, tap, well, or bottled)

If breastfeeding, number of feedings, length of time at the breast, number of wet diapers, and supplemental feedings

Favorite foods, food dislikes, food jags, food allergies, food intolerances, lack of dietary variety with regard to solids

Frequency, length, and location of feedings, meals, and snacks

Child's independence in obtaining food, including use of bottle or cup for beverages

Current and past use of oral nutritional supplements or special diets or diet consistencies

Fluid intake and bowel habits

Cultural or ethnic family eating practices

Use of complementary/alternative nutrition therapies, including restrictive diets

BOX 5.1   Key Elements of a Pediatric Diet History (cont.)

Activity level or ambulation, including physical inactivity time

Pertinent eating/feeding history

Caregiver's perception of the role of nutrition/feeding practices as they relate to the child's health condition

Caregiver's ability to recognize hunger and satiety cues

Other programs or therapies that may be providing food as a reward/therapy

Use of nonoral enteral feeding

Adapted with permission from Green Corkin K, Whittenbrook W, eds. *Academy of Nutrition and Dietetics Pocket Guide to Children with Special Health Care and Nutritional Needs.* 2nd ed. Chicago, IL: Academy of Nutrition and Dietetics; in press.[8]

Methods for Obtaining Diet Histories

Several methods are available for obtaining a diet history (see Box 5.2, pages 116 to 119).[3,4] Each method has merits and limitations. The method selected should be based on the setting, source of information, access to the information, ease of data collection, and depth of information required. Regardless of the method used, the history should include all foods, beverages, medications, and supplements consumed; the portions of each; and the time when and location where they are consumed.

BOX 5.2   Types of Diet Histories[3,4]

Diet Interview

Trained food and nutrition professional conducts a detailed interview.

Advantages:

- Comprehensive review of factors affecting dietary intake
- May be steered by the interviewer using advanced techniques (eg, motivational interviewing) to assess readiness for change

Disadvantages:

- Time consuming
- Yields higher estimated intake than 24-hour recall or food records

24-Hour Recall

Interviewer solicits recall of actual intake in the previous 24 hours or of a "typical" 24 hours from child or caregiver. (Typical 24 hours may be more appropriate if child is acutely ill.)

Advantages:

- Quick
- Easy to perform
- Provides a snapshot
- Does not require record keeping

BOX 5.2 Types of Diet Histories[3,4] (cont.)

Disadvantages:

- May not be reflective of usual intake
- Relies on recollection
- Tends to underestimate intake

3-Day Food Record

Child or caregiver is asked to record actual intake for 3 consecutive days. Client may be provided with a form to record intake or may be asked to keep a food diary. Record should include 1 weekend day to account for differing consumption patterns.

Advantages:

- Data gathered prospectively
- Includes actual (reported) amounts of food consumed
- Provides a more comprehensive picture of usual intake than 24-hour recall
- Suitable for computer analysis

Disadvantages:

- Requires record keeping by child/caregiver
- Completion of nutrition assessment delayed
- Family may change diet pattern since they know it is being monitored

Continued on next page

BOX 5.2   Types of Diet Histories[3,4] (cont.)

7-Day Food Record

Child or caregiver is asked to record actual intake for 7 consecutive days. Client may be provided with a form to record intake or may be asked to keep a food diary.

Advantages:

- Data gathered prospectively
- Provides a more comprehensive picture of usual intake than either 24-hour recall or 3-day record
- Suitable for computer analysis

Disadvantages:

- Compliance with keeping the record may be low
- Accuracy may deteriorate over time
- Intervention may be delayed

Food Frequency

Child or caregiver completes a questionnaire designed to gather data on the frequency and amount of foods eaten.

Advantages:

- Decreases time required for interview
- Can provide a more complete picture of nutrient adequacy than 24-hour recall

BOX 5.2   Types of Diet Histories[3,4] (cont.)

Disadvantages:

- Difficult to assess unique details of diet
- Overreporting of intake is common
- May not have certain cultural foods listed

Calorie Count

Used by inpatient health care facilities to document adequacy of intake. Professional staff (eg, nurse; dietetics technician, registered; and/or registered dietitian nutritionist) records actual intake at the bedside.

Advantages:

- Useful for documenting actual intake in a controlled environment
- Can provide a rough assessment of appetite, intake, and compliance with nutrition regimen

Disadvantages:

- Not representative of usual intake at home
- Accuracy limited by multiple professionals recording intake

Evaluation

Evaluation of the diet history can also be performed in a number of ways, depending on the type and extent of information needed. Intake of energy and macronutrients can be estimated using values for common portions of foods or using exchanges, which use approximate values for similar foods (see Table 5.1).[5] Computer analysis is more appropriate than estimates for assessment of micronutrient intake as well as for the precise assessment of macronutrient intake. A variety of proprietary and free software tools and applications are available for use in analyzing dietary intake data. The US Department of Agriculture (USDA) National Nutrient Database is a searchable tool that provides both macronutrient and micronutrient content of common American foods.[5]

TABLE 5.1 Energy and Protein Content of Foods Commonly Consumed by Infants and Children[5]

Food	Serving Size	Energy, kcal	Protein, g
Breastmilk	1 oz	~20[a]	0.3
Infant formula	1 oz	20	0.4
Baby Foods			
Rice cereal, dry	1 Tbsp	10	0.2
Fruit, pureed	3.5 oz pouch[b]	45–65	0.2
Vegetable, pureed	4 oz pouch[b]	30–50	0.9–4.0
Meat, chicken, strained	4 oz jar[b]	105	13.4
Dinner, turkey and vegetable, strained	4 oz jar[b]	54	2.6
Meltable solids (vegetable/fruit puffs)	32 pieces	25	<1
Grains			
Breakfast cereal, toasted oat rings	1 c	111	3.6

TABLE 5.1   Energy and Protein Content of Foods Commonly Consumed by Infants and Children[5] (cont.)

Food	Serving Size	Energy, kcal	Protein, g
Grains (cont.)			
Instant oatmeal, prepared with water	1 packet	97	4.1
Bread, white	1 slice	67	1.9
Hamburger/hotdog bun	1 small	120	4.1
Bagel, plain, 3½- to 4-in diameter	1	289	11.0
Pasta (plain, cooked macaroni, spaghetti)	½ c	111	4.1
Rice, white	½ c	97	2.3
Vegetables			
Broccoli, chopped, boiled	½ c	27	1.9
Carrots, baby, raw	1 large	5	0.1
Carrots, sliced, boiled	½ c	27	0.6
Green beans, steamed	½ c	22	1.2
Potato, baked	1 medium	145	3.1
French fries, fast food	Small	227	2.5
Fruits			
Apple	1 medium	72	0.4
Banana	1 medium	105	1.3
Grapes	½ c	55	0.6
Strawberries	½ c	24	0.5
Apple juice, 100%	4 oz	58	0.1
Grape juice, 100%	4 oz	77	0.7

Continued on next page

TABLE 5.1   Energy and Protein Content of Foods Commonly Consumed by Infants and Children[5] (cont.)

Food	Serving Size	Energy, kcal	Protein, g
Milk and Dairy Foods			
Whole milk	4 oz	73	3.9
Reduced-fat (2%) milk, protein fortified	4 oz	69	4.5
Low-fat (1%) milk, protein fortified	4 oz	59	4.8
Fat-free (skim) milk	4 oz	42	4.1
Whole milk yogurt, plain	4 oz	69	3.9
Low-fat yogurt with fruit	6 oz	163	6.5
Nonfat yogurt with fruit	8 oz	230	10.8
Cheese, cheddar	1 oz	114	7.1
Cheese, America	1 oz	106	6.3
Cheese, mozzarella, part skim	1 oz	72	6.9
Protein Foods			
Egg	1 large	78	6.3
Beef, ground, 85% lean, cooked	3 oz	218	23.6
Chicken, skinless breast, roasted	3 oz	142	26.7
Chicken nuggets	3 pieces	143	7.5
Fish, white (flounder, sole), baked	3 oz	96	20.5
Pork, boneless, panfried	3 oz	177	20.0

TABLE 5.1 Energy and Protein Content of Foods Commonly Consumed by Infants and Children[5] (cont.)

Food	Serving Size	Energy, kcal	Protein, g
Protein Foods			
Peanut butter	2 Tbsp	188	8.0
Beans, cooked	½ c	112	7.7
Fats			
Avocado	1 Tbsp	25	0
Butter or margarine	1 tsp	36	0
Vegetable oil	1 tsp	40	0
Cream cheese	1 Tbsp	51	1.1
Mayonnaise	1 Tbsp	57	0.1
Salad dressing, ranch	1 Tbsp	73	0.2
Combination Foods			
Macaroni and cheese, prepared per box	1 c	380	11.3
Pizza, plain cheese, 14-in pizzeria style	1 slice	272	11.6
Snacks, Sweets, and Beverages			
Potato chips	1 oz	155	1.9
Goldfish crackers	20	60	1.2
Pretzels	1 oz	108	2.9
Jelly	1 Tbsp	56	0
Chocolate chip cookie, 2 ¼-in diameter	1	49	0.6
Cupcake	1 small	131	1.9

Continued on next page

Food and Nutrition History

TABLE 5.1	Energy and Protein Content of Foods Commonly Consumed by Infants and Children[5] (cont.)		
Food	Serving Size	Energy, kcal	Protein, g
Snacks, Sweets, and Beverages (cont.)			
Granola bar, soft, peanut butter	1 each	119	2.9
Sandwich cookie, chocolate with cream	1 each	47	0.5
Ice cream, regular	½ c	145	2.5
Ice cream, light	½ c	125	3.6
Popsicle, 1.75 fluid oz	1 pop	12	0
Soft drink	4 oz	45	0.1
Fruit aid	4 oz	58	0
Sport drink	4 oz	31	0

[a] Approximate energy content of breastmilk for full-term infants is about 20 kcal. Energy content varies depending on the length of term, age of the infant, and from beginning to end of each feeding
[b] Infant foods are packaged in containers varying from 2 to 6 oz. Exact container size should be noted in diet history

To assess nutritional adequacy, the child's diet should be compared to the Dietary Reference Intakes (DRIs) or other credible reference standards.[6] See Chapter 8 for more information on DRIs.

Infant and Toddler Feeding Skills

During the first 3 years of life, feeding skills develop in a progressive fashion from basic sucking to adult-like feeding. This progression is accomplished through the acquisition of fine, gross, and oral-motor skills. At each point in development, the foods presented must match the infant's or toddler's skills to ensure nutritional adequacy of the diet (see Box 5.3).[7]

BOX 5.3	Physical Abilities, Eating Skills, Hunger and Fullness Cues, and Appropriate Food Textures for Infants and Toddlers[7]
Newborn	
Physical abilities:	Needs head support
Eating skills:	Baby establishes suck-swallow-breathe pattern during breastfeeding or bottle feeding
Hunger and fullness cues:	Cries or fusses to show hunger; gazes at caregiver, opens mouth during feeding, indicating desire to continue; spits out nipple or falls asleep when full; stops sucking when full

Continued on next page

BOX 5.3   Physical Abilities, Eating Skills, Hunger and Fullness Cues, and Appropriate Food Textures for Infants and Toddlers[7] (cont.)

Infant Who Can Hold Head Up

Physical abilities:	More skillful head control with support emerging
Eating skills:	Breastfeeds or bottle feeds; tongue moves forward and back to suck
Hunger and fullness cues:	Cries or fusses to show hunger; smiles, gazes at caregiver, or coos during feeding to indicate desire to continue; spits out nipple or falls asleep when full; stops sucking when full
Appropriate food textures:	Breastmilk or infant formula

Supported Sitter

Physical abilities:	Sits with help or support; on tummy, pushes up on arms with straight elbows
Eating skills:	May push food out of mouth with tongue, which gradually decreases with age; moves pureed food forward and backward in mouth with tongue to swallow; recognizes spoon and holds mouth open as spoon approaches

BOX 5.3	Physical Abilities, Eating Skills, Hunger and Fullness Cues, and Appropriate Food Textures for Infants and Toddlers[7] (cont.)
Hunger and fullness cues:	Moves head forward to reach spoon when hungry; may swipe the food toward the mouth when hungry; turns head away from spoon when full; may be distracted or notice surroundings more when full
Appropriate food textures:	Breastmilk or infant formula; infant cereals; thin pureed foods

Neuromuscular disorders, psychosocial disorders, and obstructive lesions may interfere with the development of feeding skills and result in nutrition problems. For infants and toddlers in whom a delay in feeding skills is suspected, the clinician should arrange to observe the child being fed, preferably by the caregiver. For more information about children with developmental delays, consult the *Academy of Nutrition and Dietetics Pocket Guide to Children with Special Health Care and Nutritional Needs*.[8]

Eating Patterns

Eating patterns develop and change substantially during infancy, childhood, and adolescence. Each period of development is marked by typical behaviors that may influence the potential development of nutritional abnormalities (see Box 5.4).[9-12] The clinician must be aware of these behaviors with the goal of providing anticipatory guidance to help establish healthy eating patterns. Box 5.5 (page 130) provides age-specific feeding/eating patterns to explore during the dietary assessment.[9,10,13]

BOX 5.4   Typical Feeding/Eating Behaviors for Age[9-12]

Infants

Depend entirely on caregivers to meet their needs

Have limited ability to convey hunger and fullness, requiring caregivers to be attentive to cues (eg, roots for nipple and cries or fusses to display hunger, spits out the nipple, stops sucking, or falls asleep to display fullness)

Need only breastmilk or iron-fortified infant formula for the first 6 months of life to meet their nutritional needs

Developmentally ready for the introduction of complementary foods between 4 and 6 months of age

Toddlers

Demonstrate independence in self-feeding skills and ability to communicate eating preferences and needs

Use food and eating to elicit a response from caregiver

Tend to go on food "jags" where certain foods are consumed to the exclusion of others

"Good eaters" as infants may become "fair-to-poor" eaters as toddlers

---

BOX 5.4 Typical Feeding/Eating Behaviors for Age[9-12] (cont.)

May choke on foods that are hard to control in the mouth and can be lodged in the esophagus, such as nuts, raw carrots, popcorn, and hard candy

May consume excessive amounts of juice, to the exclusion of milk, if given the opportunity

May be reluctant or fearful about trying new things

Preschoolers

Interest in eating may be unpredictable

May have a limited attention span at the table

Food selection and intake patterns are highly influenced by environmental cues, including time of day, portion sizes served, pressure to eat, food restrictions, and the eating patterns and preferences of others who are important to them, including family members and friends

May appear to eat erratically from meal to meal, but overall consumption is fairly constant

Tend to eat following a pattern similar to adults but are not capable of choosing a well-balanced diet

BOX 5.5   Age-Specific Feeding/Eating Patterns to Evaluate in the Dietary Assessment[9,10,13]

School-Age Children

Have increased freedom over food choices and increased access to less nutritious foods outside the home

Are ready to learn basic concepts about good nutrition

Develop socially, making friends who influence food choices

Typically consume roughly 10% of dietary energy in the form of fruit juices and soft drinks

Begin to make comparisons with peers in terms of body weight and shape

Influenced by media viewing

Adolescents

Have increasing independence and busy schedules

Have an increased tendency to skip meals, especially breakfast and lunch, and tend to snack, especially on candy

Eat more meals outside the home than younger children and frequently consume fast foods

Consume soft drinks, sports drinks, coffee, tea, and alcoholic beverages, replacing milk and juice

May be dissatisfied with body image, may have a desire for peer acceptance, and may participate in dieting for weight loss or the need to conform to the adolescent lifestyle

May be influenced by media viewing

May become ritualistic about eating or avoiding certain foods

May include or omit specific foods due to religion or ideology

Recommended Food Intake Patterns

Food intake patterns for infants, children, and adolescents are another set of standards against which individual intake can be assessed.

Food Intake Patterns for Infants and Toddlers

Table 5.2 outlines the typical feeding progression of foods and typical portion sizes for infants and toddlers aged 3 and younger.[14,15]

TABLE 5.2	Typical Portion Sizes and Daily Intake for Children, Aged 0 to 36[14-16] Months[14,15]	
Age, mo	**Food (Portion Size)**	**Feedings/Servings per Day**
0–4	Breastmilk or infant formula (2–4 oz)	8–12
4–6	Breastmilk or infant formula (6–8 oz)	4–6
	Infant cereal (1–2 Tbsp)	1–2
6–8	Breastmilk or infant formula (6–8 oz)	3–5
	Infant cereal (2 Tbsp)	2
	Crackers (2), bread (½ slice)	1
	Meats (2 Tbsp)	1–2

Continued on next page

TABLE 5.2   Typical Portion Sizes and Daily Intake for Children, Aged 0 to 36[14-16] Months[14,15] (cont.)

Age, mo	Food (Portion Size)	Feedings/Servings per Day
8–12	Breastmilk or infant formula (6–8 oz)	3–4
	Cheese (½ oz) or yogurt (½ c)	1
	Infant cereal (2–4 Tbsp), bread (½ slice), crackers (2), or pasta (3–4 Tbsp)	2
	Fruit or vegetable (3–4 Tbsp)	2–3
	Meat (3–4 Tbsp) or beans (¼ c)	2
	Milk (4 oz), cheese (½ oz), yogurt (½ c), or cottage cheese (¼ c)	4–5
12–36	Cereal (⅓–½ c), pasta (¼–⅓ c), rice (¼–⅓ c), bread (¼–½ slice), crackers (2)	6
	Fruits, including juice[a] (⅓ c canned or fresh chopped)	2–3
	Vegetables (¼ c)	2–3
	Meat or fish (1–3 Tbsp), egg (1), beans (¼ c)	2

[a] Limit maximum daily juice intake to 4 oz

Food Intake Patterns Defined by the US Department of Agriculture's MyPlate

The USDA food guidance system, ChooseMyPlate, along with the Dietary Guidelines for Americans, provides daily food intake patterns for individuals aged 2 years to adult based on estimated energy needs (see Box 5.6 on pages 134 and 135 and Tables 5.3 to 5.6 on pages 135 to 139).[17-19] The Choose MyPlate website (www.choose myplate.gov) includes tools to select the appropriate calorie level and daily food pattern for a particular individual.[17] It is important to recognize that these calorie levels are based on average needs and are not appropriate for determining calorie needs of individual patients in a clinical setting. See the section Estimated Energy Requirements in Chapter 8 for more information on estimating individualized energy requirements based on sex, age, weight, height, and activity level.

BOX 5.6   Choose MyPlate Food Groups[19]

Grains include all foods made from wheat, rice, oats, corn-meal, barley, and other cereal grains (eg, bread, pasta, oatmeal, breakfast cereals, tortillas, and grits). Grains can be divided into whole grains, those that retain the entire grain kernel, and refined grains, those that have been milled (ie, removing the germ and bran). *At least half of all grains consumed should be whole grains.* In general, 1 slice of bread, 1 cup of ready-to-eat cereal, or ½ cup of cooked rice, pasta, or cooked cereal can be considered an ounce equivalent from the grains group.

Fruits include all fresh, frozen, canned, and dried fruits, as well as fruit juices. In general, 1 cup of fruit, 1 cup of 100% fruit juice, or ½ cup of dried fruit can be considered as 1 cup from the fruit group.

Vegetables include all fresh, frozen, canned, and dried vegetables, as well as vegetable juices. In general, 1 cup of raw or cooked vegetables, 1 cup of vegetable juice, or 2 cups of raw leafy greens can be considered as 1 cup from the vegetables group. Vegetables are organized in five subgroups based on their nutrient content. Weekly recommendations for each subgroup are provided.

Protein foods include foods made from meat, poultry, fish, dry beans or peas, eggs, nuts, and seeds. In general, 1 oz of lean meat, poultry, or fish, 1 egg, 1 Tbsp peanut butter, ¼ cup cooked dry beans, or ½ oz of nuts or seeds can be considered an ounce equivalent from the meat and beans group.

BOX 5.6 Choose MyPlate Food Groups[19] (cont.)

Dairy includes all fluid milk products and foods made from milk that retain their calcium content, such as yogurt and cheese. Calcium-fortified soymilk (soy beverage) is also part of this group. Foods made from milk that have little or no calcium, such as cream cheese, cream, and butter, are not part of the group. For children aged 2 years and older, most dairy group choices should be nonfat or low fat. In general, 1 cup of milk, yogurt, or soymilk (soy beverage), 1 ½ oz of natural cheese, or 2 oz of processed cheese can be considered as 1 cup from the milk group.

Oils include fats from many different plants and from fish that are liquid at room temperature, such as canola, corn olive, soybean, and sunflower oil. Some foods are naturally high in oils, such as nuts, olives, some fish, and avocados. Foods that are mainly oily, such as mayonnaise, certain salad dressings, and soft margarine with no *trans* fat, are part of this group.

TABLE 5.3 US Department of Agriculture Estimated Daily Calorie Requirements for Boys and Girls[a]

| Age, y | Activity Level[b] | | |
	Sedentary	Moderately Active	Active
2	Boys and girls: 1,000	Boys and girls: 1,000	Boys and girls: 1,000
3	Boys: 1,200 Girls: 1,000	Boys: 1,400 Girls: 1,200	Boys: 1,400 Girls: 1,400

Continued on next page

Food and Nutrition History

TABLE 5.3   US Department of Agriculture Estimated Daily Calorie Requirements for Boys and Girls[a] (cont.)

Activity Level[b]		
Age, y	Sedentary	Moderately Active	Active
4	Boys: 1,200 Girls: 1,200	Boys: 1,400 Girls: 1,400	Boys: 1,600 Girls: 1,400
5	Boys: 1,200 Girls: 1,200	Boys: 1,400 Girls: 1,400	Boys: 1,600 Girls: 1,600
6	Boys: 1,400 Girls: 1,200	Boys: 1,600 Girls: 1,400	Boys: 1,800 Girls: 1,600
7	Boys: 1,400 Girls: 1,200	Boys: 1,600 Girls: 1,600	Boys: 1,800 Girls: 1,800
8	Boys: 1,400 Girls: 1,400	Boys: 1,600 Girls: 1,600	Boys: 2,000 Girls: 1,800
9	Boys: 1,600 Girls: 1,400	Boys: 1,800 Girls: 1,600	Boys: 2,000 Girls: 1,800
10	Boys: 1,600 Girls: 1,400	Boys: 1,800 Girls: 1,800	Boys: 2,200 Girls: 2,000
11	Boys: 1,800 Girls: 1,600	Boys: 2,000 Girls: 1,800	Boys: 2,200 Girls: 2,000
12	Boys: 1,800 Girls: 1,600	Boys: 2,200 Girls: 2,000	Boys: 2,400 Girls: 2,200
13	Boys: 2,000 Girls: 1,600	Boys: 2,200 Girls: 2,000	Boys: 2,600 Girls: 2,200
14	Boys: 2,000 Girls: 1,800	Boys: 2,400 Girls: 2,000	Boys: 2,800 Girls: 2,400

TABLE 5.3 US Department of Agriculture Estimated Daily Calorie Requirements for Boys and Girls[a] (cont.)

Activity Level[b]			
Age, y	Sedentary	Moderately Active	Active
15	Boys: 2,200	Boys: 2,600	Boys: 3,000
	Girls: 1,800	Girls: 2,000	Girls: 2,400
16–18	Boys: 2,400	Boys: 2,800	Boys: 3,200
	Girls: 1,800	Girls: 2,000	Girls: 2,400

[a] Estimates are based on Estimated Energy Requirement (EER) equations, using reference heights (average) and reference weights (healthy) for each age-gender group (see Chapter 8 for more information on EER). The estimates are rounded to the nearest 200 calories for assignment to a US Department of Agriculture Daily Checklist. An individual's calorie needs may be higher or lower than these average estimates

[b] *Sedentary* means a lifestyle that includes only the light physical activity associated with typical day-to-day life. *Moderately active* means a lifestyle that includes physical activity equivalent to walking about 1.5 to 3 miles per day at 3 to 4 miles per hour, in addition to the light physical activity associated with typical day-to-day life. *Active* means a lifestyle that includes physical activity equivalent to walking more than 3 miles per day at 3 to 4 miles per hour in addition to the light physical activity associated with typical day-to-day life

Adapted from US Department of Health and Human Services and US Department of Agriculture. *2015-2020 Dietary Guidelines for Americans.* 8th ed. Washington, DC: US Department of Health and Human Services; 2015.[18]

TABLE 5.4 MyPlate Plan: 1,000 to 1,600 kcal/d[a]

Food Group	1,000 Calorie	1,200 Calorie	1,400 Calorie	1,600 Calorie
Fruits	1 c	1 c	1½ c	1½ c
Vegetables	1 c	1½ c	1½ c	2 c
Grains	3 oz	4 oz	5 oz	5 oz
Protein foods	2 oz	3 oz	4 oz	5 oz
Dairy	2 c	2½ c	2½ c	2½ c

Continued on next page

TABLE 5.4　MyPlate Plan: 1,000 to 1,600 kcal/d[a] (cont.)

Food Group	1,000 Calorie	1,200 Calorie	1,400 Calorie	1,600 Calorie
LIMIT:				
Sodium	<1,500 mg	<1,500 mg	<1,500 mg	<1,900 mg
Saturated fats	<11 g	<13 g	<16 g	<18 g
Added sugar	<25 g	<30 g	<35 g	<40 g

[a] Refer to Box 5.6 for definitions of food groups and portion equivalents
Adapted from US Department of Agriculture. Choose MyPlate website. www.choose myplate.gov/MyPlatePlan. Accessed August 16, 2018.[19]

TABLE 5.5　MyPlate Plan: 1,800 to 2,400 kcal/d[a]

Food Group	1,800 Calorie	2,000 Calorie	2,200 Calorie	2,400 Calorie
Fruits	1½ c	2 c	2 c	2 c
Vegetables	2½ c	2½ c	3 c	3 c
Grains	6 oz	6 oz	7 oz	8 oz
Protein foods	5 oz	5½ oz	6 oz	6½ oz
Dairy	2½ c	2½ c	3 c	3 c
LIMIT:				
Sodium	<1,900 mg	<1,900 mg	<2,200 mg	<2,200 mg
Saturated fats	<20 g	<22 g	<24 g	<27 g
Added sugar	<45 g	<50 g	<55 g	<60 g

[a] Refer to Box 5.6 for definitions of food groups and portion equivalents.
Adapted from US Department of Agriculture. MyPlate Plan. www.choosemyplate.gov/MyPlatePlan. Accessed August 16, 2018.[19]

Food Group	2,600 Calorie	2,800 Calorie	3,000 Calorie	3,200 Calorie
Fruits	2 c	2½ c	2½ c	2½ c
Vegetables	3½ c	3½ c	4 c	4 c
Grains	9 oz	10 oz	10 oz	10 oz
Protein foods	6½ oz	7 oz	7 oz	7 oz
Dairy	3 c	3 c	3 c	3 c
LIMIT:				
Sodium	<2,200 mg	<2,200 mg	<2,200 mg	<2,300 mg
Saturated fats	<29 g	<31 g	<33 g	<36 g
Added sugar	<65 g	<70 g	<75 g	<80 g

TABLE 5.6   MyPlate Daily Checklist: 2,600 to 2,800 kcal/d[a]

[a]Refer to Box 5.6 for definitions of food groups and portion equivalents

Adapted from US Department of Agriculture. Choose MyPlate website. www.choose myplate.gov/MyPlatePlan. Accessed August 16, 2018.[19]

Portion Sizes for Toddlers, Preschoolers, and School-Age Children

The USDA food intake patterns provide the total amount of each food group to be consumed in a day (eg, 1 cup of fruit; 5 oz equivalents of grains).[17-19] When dividing these amounts into portions, it is important to note that portion sizes for toddlers, preschoolers, and school-aged children are generally smaller than those for adults, and they increase with age. A general rule for toddler and preschool children is to offer 1 Tbsp of each food per year of the child's age; more can be provided based on the child's appetite.[10] Portion sizes for older school-aged children and adolescents are generally the same as those for adults.[11] When using the USDA food intake patterns, the recommended daily amount should be divided into the appropriate number of child-size portions, based on age. For example, if 2 cups of dairy are recommended and the appropriate portion size of milk for the child's age is a ½ cup, then four portions of milk meet the daily requirement. Table 5.7 provides examples of appropriate portion sizes for children from 2 to 12 years of age.

TABLE 5.7	Portion Sizes for Children Aged 2 to 12 Years[10,17]		
Food Group	**2–3 y**	**4–6 y**	**7–12 y**
Fruits			
Raw[a]	½–1 small piece	½–1 small piece	1 medium piece
Canned	2–3 Tbsp	4–6 Tbsp	¼–½ c
Juice	3–4 oz	4 oz	4 oz
Vegetables			
Cooked	2–3 Tbsp	4–6 Tbsp	¼–½ c
Raw[a]	Few pieces	Few pieces	Several pieces
Grains			
Whole grain or enriched bread	½–1 slice	1 slice	1 slice
Whole grain or enriched buns, bagels, or English muffins	¼–½	½	½

TABLE 5.7	Portion Sizes for Children Aged 2 to 12 Years[10,17] (cont.)		
Food Group	**2–3 y**	**4–6 y**	**7–12 y**
Grains			
Pasta or rice	½–1 c	½ c	½ c
Cooked cereal	¼–½ c	½ c	½–1 c
Dry cereal	½–1 c	1 c	1 c
Protein Foods			
Meat, poultry, fish, eggs, peanut butter, or dry beans[b]	1–2 oz	1–2 oz	2 oz
Oils	4 tsp	4–5 tsp	4–6 tsp
Dairy			
Milk, yogurt, and cheese[c]	½ c (4 oz)	½–¾ c (4–6 oz)	½–1 c (4–8 oz)

[a] May present a risk for choking to young children or those with delayed oral motor skills
[b] 1 egg = 1 oz; 2 Tbsp peanut butter = 1 oz; 4 Tbsp dry beans = 1 oz
[c] ½–¾ oz cheese = ½ cup fluid milk

References

1. Nevin-Folino N, Ogata BN, Charney PJ, et al. Academy of Nutrition and Dietetics: Revised 2015 Standards of Practice and Standards of Professional Performance for Registered Dietitian Nutritionist (Competent, Proficient, and Expert) in Pediatric Nutrition. *J Acad Nutr Diet*. 2015;115:451-460.

2. Weston SC, Murray P. Diet and nutrition. In: DeVore J, Shotton A, eds. *Academy of Nutrition and Dietetics Pocket Guide to Children with Special Health Care and Nutritional Needs*. Chicago, IL: Academy of Nutrition and Dietetics; 2012:22-75.

3. Bessler S. Nutritional assessment. In: Samour PQ, King K, eds. *Handbook of Pediatric Nutrition.* 4th ed. Sudbury, MA: Jones and Bartlett; 2012:35-52.

4. Olsen IE, Mascarenhas MR, Stallings VA. Clinical assessment of nutritional status. In: Walker WA, Watkins JB, Duggan C, eds. *Nutrition in Pediatrics.* 3rd ed. Hamilton, ON: BC Decker; 2003:6-16.

5. Nutrient Data Laboratory, United States Department of Agriculture. USDA National Nutrient Database for Windows Search Software. https://ndb.nal.usda.gov/ndb. Accessed January 25, 2018.

6. Academy of Nutrition and Dietetics. *Abridged Nutrition Care Process Terminology (NCPT) Reference Manual: Standardized Terminology for the Nutrition Care Process.* Chicago, IL: Academy of Nutrition and Dietetics; 2017:7.

7. Butte N, Cobb K, Dwyer J, Graney L, Heird W, Rickard K. The start healthy feeding guidelines for infants and toddlers. *J Am Diet Assoc.* 2004;104:442-454.

8. Green Corkin K, Whittenbrook W, eds. *Academy of Nutrition and Dietetics Pocket Guide to Children with Special Health Care and Nutritional Needs.* 2nd ed. Chicago, IL: Academy of Nutrition and Dietetics; in press.

9. Complementary feeding. In: Kleinman RE, Greer FR, eds. *Pediatric Nutrition Handbook.* 7th ed. Elk Grove Village, IL: American Academy of Pediatrics; 2014:123-139.

10. Feeding the child. In: Kleinman RE, Greer FR, eds. *Pediatric Nutrition Handbook.* 7th ed. Elk Grove Village, IL: American Academy of Pediatrics; 2014:143-173.

11. Adolescent nutrition. In: Kleinman RE, Greer FR, eds. *Pediatric Nutrition Handbook.* 7th ed. Elk Grove Village, IL: American Academy of Pediatrics; 2014:175-187.

12. Lucas B, Ogata B, Feucht S. Normal nutrition from infancy through adolescence. In: Samour PQ, King K, eds. *Handbook of Pediatric Nutrition*. 4th ed. Boston, MA: Jones and Bartlett; 2012:103-126.

13. American Academy of Pediatrics. *Bright Futures Nutrition*. 3rd ed. http://brightfutures.aap.org/nutrition_3rd_Edition .html. Accessed January 25, 2018.

14. Academy of Nutrition and Dietetics Pediatric Nutrition Care Manual. Normal nutrition: full-term infants. www.nutritioncaremanual.org/category.cfm?ncm_category _id=12&ncm_heading=. Accessed January 25, 2018.

15. Academy of Nutrition and Dietetics Pediatric Nutrition Care Manual. Normal nutrition: toddlers. www.nutrition caremanual.org/category.cfm?ncm_category_id=12&ncm _heading=. Accessed January 25, 2018.

16. Heyman MB, Abrams SA, Section on Gastroenterology, Hepatology and Nutrition, Nutrition Committee, Committed on Nutrition. Fruit juice in infants, children and adolescents: current recommendations. *Pediatrics*. 2017;139(6): e20170967. http://pediatrics.aappublications.org /content/139/6/e20170967. Accessed May 22, 2019.

17. US Department of Agriculture. Choose MyPlate website. www.choosemyplate.gov. Accessed January 25, 2018.

18. US Department of Health and Human Services and US Department of Agriculture. *2015-2020 Dietary Guidelines for Americans*. 8th edition. Washington, DC: US Department of Health and Human Services; 2015. https://health.gov /dietaryguidelines/2015. Accessed January 25, 2018.

19. US Department of Agriculture. MyPlate Plan. Choose MyPlate website. www.choosemyplate.gov/MyPlatePlan. Accessed August 16, 2018.

CHAPTER 6

Nutrition-Focused Physical Examination

A thorough nutrition-focused physical examination (NFPE) can reveal signs and symptoms of nutrient deficiencies or excesses, which may then be confirmed by further objective testing. Because of the rapid timeframe in which an infant or child may become malnourished, completing an NFPE is an important step in the assessment process that can lead to earlier diagnosis of malnutrition.[1] See Chapter 3 for criteria to identify pediatric malnutrition.

The NFPE involves a complete physical assessment of the infant, child, or adolescent, system by system. This can be performed by any appropriately trained health care professional, including a registered dietitian nutritionist, a nurse, or a physician.[2] The Academy of Nutrition and Dietetics has developed a Nutrition Focused Physical Exam Hands-On Training Workshop for registered dietitian nutritionists; visit the Academy of Nutrition and Dietetics website (www.eatrightPRO .org/NFPE) for more information.

Many nutrition-related signs and symptoms found during the exam can later be more objectively confirmed with laboratory assessment (see Chapter 7). Boxes 6.1 to 6.11 (pages 145 to 155) outline possible exam findings, organized by system and possible nutrition-related causes of those findings; suspected malnutrition should be confirmed with other objective measures (see Chapter 3).

BOX 6.1 Skin Examination[2-5]	
Signs	**Possible Nutrition-Related Causes**
Elastic, firm; no lesions, rashes, or hyperpigmentation	Adequate/appropriate nutrition
Acanthosis nigricans (hyperpigmentation in skin folds)	Insulin resistance due to obesity
Decreased subcutaneous tissue	Prolonged protein-calorie deficit
Delayed wound healing	Vitamin C, zinc, or protein deficiency
Dermatitis (generalized)	Zinc deficiency, niacin deficiency

Continued on next page

NFPE

BOX 6.1 Skin Examination[2-5] (cont.)	
Signs	**Possible Nutrition-Related Causes**
Dryness	Vitamin A deficiency; insufficient essential and unsaturated fatty acids
Edema	Protein-calorie deficiency
Follicular hyperkeratosis	Vitamin A, vitamin C deficiency
Hyperpigmentation	Vitamin B-12, folic acid, or niacin deficiency
Orange/yellow pigmentation	Beta carotene excess
Pallor	Iron, vitamin B-12, vitamin C, folic acid, and vitamin B-6 deficiency
Poor skin turgor	Insufficient water, sodium
Petechiae	Vitamin C, vitamin K deficiency
Psoriasis	Biotin deficiency
Purpura	Vitamin C, vitamin K deficiency; vitamin E excess
Swollen red pigmentation (pellagrous dermatosis) in sun-exposed areas of skin	Niacin deficiency or secondary vitamin B-6 deficiency

BOX 6.2 Hair and Nail Examination[2-5]

Signs	Possible Nutrition-Related Causes
Hair	
Shiny, firm, elastic hair	Adequate/appropriate nutrition
Alopecia	Protein, iron, zinc, or biotin deficiency
Corkscrew-shaped hair	Vitamin C deficiency
Depigmentation or other color changes	Protein-calorie, copper, manganese, or selenium deficiency
Dull, dry, thin, brittle, sparse, easily plucked hair	Protein-calorie or essential fatty acid deficiency
Lanugo (fine, soft hair covering the body)	Calorie deficiency
Nails	
Ridges in nails	Central ridges: iron, folic acid, or protein deficiency
	Transverse ridges: zinc, protein, or calcium deficiency
Soft, brittle, or weak nails	Protein-calorie or magnesium deficiency; vitamin A, selenium excess
Koilonychias (spoon-shaped nails)	Iron or protein deficiency

BOX 6.3 Head and Neck Examination[2-5]

Signs	Possible Nutrition-Related Causes
Head	
Head evenly molded, with occipital prominence; facial features symmetric	Adequate/appropriate nutrition
Hard, tender lumps in occipital region, bulging fontanelle	Vitamin A excess
Headache	Thiamin excess, vitamin A excess
Skull flattened, frontal bones prominent	Vitamin D deficiency
Sunken fontanelle	Dehydration
Sutures fused by 12–18 months	Adequate/appropriate nutrition
Suture fusion delayed	Vitamin D deficiency
Neck	
Thyroid gland not obvious to inspection, palpable in midline	Adequate/appropriate nutrition
Thyroid gland enlarged, obvious to inspection	Iodine deficiency

BOX 6.4 Eye Examination[2-5]

Signs	Possible Nutrition-Related Causes
Clear, bright, shiny eyes; membranes pink and moist; adequate night vision	Adequate/appropriate nutrition
Dull, soft cornea; white or gray spots on cornea (Bitot's spots)	Vitamin A deficiency
Inflammation of eyelids (angular blepharitis)	Riboflavin, biotin, vitamin B-6, or zinc deficiency
Pale conjunctiva	Iron, vitamin B-6, vitamin B-12, folic acid, or copper deficiency
Night blindness	Vitamin A deficiency
Redness, fissuring at corners of eyes (angular palpebritis)	Niacin, riboflavin, vitamin B-6, or iron deficiency
Xanthelasmas	Hyperlipidemia

BOX 6.5   Nose, Mouth/Lip, and Tongue Examination[2-5]

Signs	Possible Nutrition-Related Causes
Nose	
Smooth, intact nasal angle	Adequate/appropriate nutrition
Cracks, irritation at nasal angle	Niacin deficiency; vitamin A excess
Mouth/Lips	
Smooth, moist lips, no edema	Adequate/appropriate nutrition and hydration
Angular fissures, redness, and edema (angular stomatitis or cheilitis)	Riboflavin, niacin, iron, vitamin B-6, or vitamin B-12 deficiency; vitamin A excess
Tongue	
Deep-pink tongue, papillae visible, moist, taste sensation, no edema	Adequate/appropriate nutrition
Decreased taste	Zinc deficiency
Magenta coloration, soreness, burning	Riboflavin deficiency

BOX 6.5   Nose, Mouth/Lip, and Tongue Examination[2-5] (cont.)

Signs	Possible Nutrition-Related Causes
Paleness	Vitamin B-12, folic acid, or iron deficiency
Raw, beefy-red, swollen sore	Folic acid or niacin deficiency
Red, swollen, sore, smooth (glossitis)	Riboflavin, folic acid, niacin, vitamin B-6, vitamin B-12, or iron deficiency

BOX 6.6   Gum and Teeth Examination[2-5]

Signs	Possible Nutrition-Related Causes
Gums	
Firm, coral color	Adequate/appropriate nutrition
Spongy, bleed easily, receding	Vitamin C deficiency
Reddened gingival	Vitamin A excess
Teeth	
White, smooth, free of spots or pits	Adequate/appropriate nutrition
Caries	Excess carbohydrates, insufficient fluoride, vitamin D deficiency

NFPE

Continued on next page

BOX 6.6 Gum and Teeth Examination[2-5] (cont.)	
Signs	**Possible Nutrition-Related Causes**
Teeth	
Defective enamel	Insufficient vitamin A, vitamin C, calcium, or phosphorous
Mottled enamel, brown spots, pits	Excess fluoride

BOX 6.7 Cardiovascular System Examination[2-5]	
Signs	**Possible Nutrition-Related Causes**
Pulse and blood pressure within normal limits for age	Adequate/appropriate nutrition
Arrhythmia	Insufficient magnesium or potassium; niacin or potassium excess
Decreased blood pressure	Insufficient thiamin, dehydration
Palpitations	Insufficient thiamin
Rapid pulse	Insufficient potassium, dehydration

BOX 6.8 Gastrointestinal Examination[2-5]

Signs	Possible Nutrition-Related Causes
Bowel habits normal for age	Adequate/appropriate nutrition
Constipation	Inadequate intake of high-fiber foods or fluids; excess calcium
Diarrhea	Excess intake of juice; high consumption of fresh fruit; vitamin B-12 or vitamin B-6 deficiency; insufficient niacin; vitamin C excess

BOX 6.9 Musculoskeletal Examination[2-5]

Signs	Possible Nutrition-Related Causes
Muscles firm and well developed, joints flexible and pain free, extremities symmetric and straight, spinal nerves normal	Adequate/appropriate nutrition
Beading on ribs	Vitamin C or vitamin D deficiency
Bleeding into joints, pain	Vitamin C deficiency

NFPE

Continued on next page

BOX 6.9   Musculoskeletal Examination[2-5] (cont.)

Signs	Possible Nutrition-Related Causes
Calf tenderness, foot drop	Thiamin deficiency
Demineralization of bone	Calcium, phosphorus, or vitamin D deficiency; vitamin A excess
Knock-knee, bow-leg, epiphyseal enlargement	Vitamin D deficiency
Muscles atrophied, dependent edema	Protein-calorie deficiency
Muscle cramps	Calcium, vitamin D, chloride, sodium, potassium, or magnesium deficiency; dehydration
Muscle pain	Biotin or vitamin D deficiency
Muscle twitching (tetany)	Calcium, vitamin D, or magnesium deficiency; magnesium or vitamin B-6 excess
Pins and needles (peripheral neuropathy)	Folic acid, vitamin B-6, pantothenic acid, vitamin B-12, thiamin, or phosphate deficiency; vitamin B-6 toxicity

BOX 6.10   Neurological System Examination[2-5]

Signs	Possible Nutrition-Related Causes
Behavior alert and responsive, intact muscle innervation	Adequate/appropriate nutrition
Convulsions	Thiamin, vitamin B-6, vitamin D, or calcium deficiency; phosphorus excess
Diminished reflexes	Thiamin deficiency
Listlessness, irritability, lethargy	Protein-calorie, thiamin, niacin, iron, or vitamin B-6 deficiency
Tetany	Magnesium deficiency
Unsteadiness, numbness in hands and feet	Vitamin B-6 excess

BOX 6.11   Sexual Maturation Examination[2-5]

Signs	Possible Nutrition-Related Causes
Age-appropriate sexual development	Adequate/appropriate nutrition
Delayed sexual maturation	Vitamin A, vitamin D, or protein-calorie deficiency

NFPE

References

1. Corkins KG. Nutrition-focused physical examination in pediatric patients. *Nutr Clin Pract*. 2015;30:203-209.

2. Secker DJ, JeeJeebhoy KN. How to perform subjective global nutrition assessment in children. *J Acad Nutr Diet*. 2012;112:424-431.

3. Mordarski B, Wolff J, eds. *Pediatric Nutrition Focused Physical Exam Pocket Guide*. Chicago, IL: Academy of Nutrition and Dietetics; 2015.

4. Engel J. *Mosby Pocket Guide to Pediatric Assessment*. 5th ed. St. Louis, MO: Mosby; 2006.

5. Zemel BS, Maqbool A, Olsen IE. Clinical assessment of nutritional status. In: Duggan C, Watkins JB, Koletzko B, Walker WA, eds. *Nutrition in Pediatrics: Basic Science, Clinical Applications*. 5th ed. Shelton, CT: People's Medical Publishing House-USA; 2016.

CHAPTER 7

Biochemical Data, Medical Tests, and Medical Procedures

When available, biochemical data, medical tests, and medical procedures can be used for the following:

- screening for malnutrition
- evaluation of nutritional status
- diagnosis of insufficient intakes of specific nutrients
- monitoring of nutritional rehabilitation

Use and Interpretation of Biochemical Data

Laboratory assessment is essential for determining hematologic, protein, and hydration status, as well as specific nutrient deficiencies.[1] Biochemical analyses are most often performed on blood, urine, or stool specimens. However, breath, hair, nails, or other body tissues may also be used.

The interpretation of results must take into consideration laboratory-specific reference standards for age, current and past medical status, and both nutrition and nonnutrition factors that alter biochemical data. The value of data to be gained from each test should be weighed against both the invasiveness of the procedure and its cost; laboratory testing should be used thoughtfully and selectively. In an evaluation of the ability of 16 nutrition-related serum biomarkers to predict clinical outcomes of critically ill children, none of the tests revealed any associations.[2]

Protein Values and Nutritional Status

Albumin has been widely used as a marker of nutritional status. However, it should be used with caution because its relatively long half-life (approximately 20 days) and ability to be affected by other disease states limit its usefulness.[3] Serum albumin levels do not reflect recent dietary intake, and results may even be normal in patients with severe protein-energy malnutrition.[3] Serum albumin levels are most useful in monitoring changes over time and are not generally helpful as single-time indicators of nutritional status for individuals in inpatient care.

Other serum proteins, including prealbumin (transthyretin), retinol-binding protein, and transferrin, have shorter half-lives. However, they can also be affected by energy restriction, iron deficiency, renal function, inflammation, or infection, as well as by protein intake.[1,3]

Table 7.1 presents normal laboratory values for serum protein. Table 7.2 (page 160) presents normal laboratory values for urine protein.[1]

TABLE 7.1	Selected Serum Protein Tests and Normal Values[1]	
Laboratory Test	**Normal Values**	
Albumin, serum, g/dL	0–6 d:	2.6–3.6
	6–30 d:	2.8–4.0
	1–6 mo:	3.1–4.2
	7–11 mo:	3.3–4.3
	1–3 y:	3.5–4.6
	4–6 y:	3.5–5.2
	7–19 y:	3.7–5.6
	20+ y:	3.5–5.0
Blood urea nitrogen, mg/dL	0–2 y:	2.0–19.0
	3–12 y:	5.0–17.0
	13–18 y:	7.0–18.0
	19–20 y:	8.0–21.0

Continued on next page

TABLE 7.1 Selected Serum Protein Tests and Normal Values[1] (cont.)

Laboratory Test	Normal Values	
Prealbumin, mg/dL	0–11 mo:	6.0–12.0
	1–5 y:	14.0–30.0
	6–9 y:	15.0–33.0
	10–13 y:	20.0–36.0
	≥14 y:	22.0–45.0
Retinol binding protein, mg/dL	3.0–6.0	
Transferrin, mg/dL	180–370	

TABLE 7.2 Selected Urine Protein Tests and Normal Values[1]

Laboratory Test	Normal Values	
3-Methyl histidine, nmol/mg creatinine	1–6 d:	81–384
	7 d to 8 wk:	75–430
	9 wk to 12 mo:	142–377
	1–3 y:	134–647
	≥4 y:	93–323
Creatinine (24 h), mg/dL	3–8 y:	140–700
	9–12 y:	300–1,300
	13–17 y, males:	500–2,300
	13–17 y, females:	400–1,600
Creatinine/height index	>0.9	

Laboratory Testing of Vitamin and Mineral Levels

When indicated by patient history or clinical examination, testing is available to assess levels of minerals, such as calcium, magnesium, phosphorous, iodine, copper, and selenium. Although levels can be measured for most vitamins and other minerals, tests may be expensive and not readily available, making routine use impractical. Refer to Tables 7.3 and 7.4 (pages 161 to 166) for laboratory tests and normal values for selected vitamins and minerals.[1,4-6]

TABLE 7.3	Laboratory Tests and Normal Values for Selected Vitamins[1,4]		
Nutrient	**Laboratory Tests**	**Normal Values**	
Vitamin A	Serum or plasma retinol, mcg/dL	0–1 mo:	18–50
		2 mo to 12 y:	20–50
		13–17 y:	26–70
		≥18 y:	30–120
Vitamin D	25-Hydroxyvitamin-D[a], ng/mL	>20	
	1,25-OH-D3, ng/mL	15–75	
Vitamin E	Serum or plasma alpha tocopherol, mg/dL	0–1 mo:	1.0–3.5
		2–5 mo:	2.0–6.0

Continued on next page

TABLE 7.3 Laboratory Tests and Normal Values for Selected Vitamins[1,4] (cont.)

Nutrient	Laboratory Tests	Normal Values	
		6–12 mo:	3.5–8.0
		2–12 y:	5.5–9.0
		≥13 y:	5.5–18.0
Vitamin K	Prothrombin time, s	0–5 mo:	NA
		≥6 mo:	11.7–13.2
Thiamin	Red blood cell transketolase stimulation, %	<15	
Vitamin B-6	Serum pyridoxal phosphate is most commonly done, but no single test is universally accepted		
Vitamin B-12	Serum vitamin B-12, pg/mL	200–900	
	Absorption test	Excretion of more than 7.5% of ingested labeled vitamin B-12	
Folic acid[b]	Serum folate, ng/mL	>6–7	
	Red blood cell folate, ng/mL	>140–160	
Vitamin C	Plasma level, mg/dL	0.2–2.0	

[a] Preferred test to screen for vitamin D deficiency
[b] Serum folate reflects status unless intake recently increased or decreased. Red blood cell folate is a better reflection of tissue stores than serum folate

TABLE 7.4 Laboratory Tests and Normal Values for Selected Minerals[1,5,6]

Nutrient	Laboratory Tests	Normal Values	
Calcium[a]	Serum total calcium, mg/dL	Newborn:	6.9–9.4
		0–1 wk:	8.0–11.4
		1–2 wk:	8.0–11.2
		2–4 wk:	9.3–10.9
		1 mo:	9.3–10.7
		2 mo:	9.3–10.6
		3–4 mo:	9.2–10.5
		5–11 mo:	9.2–10.4
		1–3 y:	8.7–9.8
		4–20 y:	8.8–10.1
	Serum ionized calcium, mg/dL	4.48–4.92	
Copper	Serum copper, mcg/dL	0–6 mo:	20–70
		7 mo to 18 y:	90–190
		≥19 y:	70–140, males; 80–155, females
Iron[b]	Hematocrit, %	Newborn:	42.0–60.0
		1–29 d:	45.0–65.0
		1–2 mo:	31.0–55.0
		3–5 mo:	29.0–41.0
		6 mo to 1 y:	33.0–39.0
		2–5 y:	34.0–40.0
		6–11 y:	35.0–45.0

Continued on next page

TABLE 7.4 Laboratory Tests and Normal Values for Selected Minerals[1,5,6] (cont.)

Nutrient	Laboratory Tests	Normal Values	
Iron (cont.)		12–17 y:	37.0–49.0, males 36.0–46.0, females
		≥18 y:	41.0–52.0 males 36.0–46.0, females
	Hemoglobin,[c] g/dL	Newborn:	13.5–19.5
		1–29 d:	14.5–22.0
		1–2 mo:	10.0–18.0
		3–5 mo:	9.5–13.5
		6 mo to 1 y:	10.5–13.5
		2–5 y:	11.5–13.5
		6–11 y:	11.5–15.5
		12–17 y:	13.0–16.0, males 12.0–16.0, females
		≥18 y:	13.5–17.0, males 12.0–16.0, females
	Serum ferritin,[d] ng/mL	0–6 mo:	6–400, males 6–430, females
		7 mo to 2 y:	12–57, males 12–60, females
		3–14 y:	14–80, males 12–73 females

TABLE 7.4 Laboratory Tests and Normal Values for Selected Minerals[1,5,6] (cont.)

Nutrient	Laboratory Tests	Normal Values	
Iron (cont.)		15–19 y:	20–155, males 12–90 females
		20–29 y:	38–270, males 12–144 males
	Serum iron, mcg/dL	0–6 wk:	100–250
		7 wk to 11 mo:	40–100
		1–10 y:	50–120
		≥11 y	50–170, males 30–160, females
	Serum total iron-binding capacity, mcg/dL	0–2 mo:	59–175
		3 mo to 17 y:	250–400
		≥18 y:	240–450
	Serum transferrin saturation, % Concentration, mg/dL	All ages: All ages:	20–50 180–370
	Erythrocyte protoporphyrin, mcg/dL	All ages:	0–35
Magnesium	Serum magnesium, mg/dL	0–20 y:	1.5–2.5
Phosphorus	Serum phosphate, mg/dL	0–11 mo:	4.8–8.2
		1–3 y:	3.8–6.5
		4–6 y:	4.1–5.4

Continued on next page

TABLE 7.4	Laboratory Tests and Normal Values for Selected Minerals[1,5,6] (cont.)	
Nutrient	**Laboratory Tests**	**Normal Values**
Phosphorus (cont.)		7–11 y:	3.7–5.6
		12–13 y:	3.3–5.4
		14–15 y:	2.9–5.4
		16–20 y:	2.7–4.7
Selenium	Serum selenium, mcg/L	All ages:	23–190
Zinc	Serum zinc,[e] mcg/dL	0–16 y:	66–144
		≥17 y:	75–291, males; 65–256, females

[a] Serum calcium is not reflective of bone calcium status

[b] There is no *single* measure available to fully characterize iron status

[c] Hemoglobin should be used to screen for deficiency at 12 months of age. If hemoglobin is <11.0 g/dL, either serum ferritin *and* C-reactive protein *or* reticulocyte hemoglobin concentration should be evaluated

[d] Serum ferritin level may be elevated with infection, liver disease, malignancy, or chronic inflammation; simultaneous measurement of C-reactive protein is required

[e] Serum zinc level may be affected by stress, growth rate, or infection

Screening and Assessment for Vitamin D Deficiency

Vitamin D deficiency seems to be increasing in the United States. See Chapter 8 for further discussion of vitamin D requirements. The prevalence of vitamin D deficiency among American children aged 6 to 18 years is reported to be 21% among healthy weight children, 29%

among overweight children, 34% among obese children, and 49% among severely obese children.[7]

While there is increased awareness of low dietary vitamin D in the United States, screening for vitamin D deficiency is recommended only in children and adolescents with certain conditions (eg, lower bone mass) or in whom multiple low-impact bone fractures have occurred.[8] Routine screening of healthy and obese children is not recommended.

The preferred test for measuring vitamin D status is serum 25-hydroxyvitamin D. (See Table 7.3 on pages 161 and 162 for normal values.)

Screening and Assessment for Nutritional Anemias

Iron-Deficiency Anemia

Iron-deficiency anemia is the most common nutrient deficiency disease worldwide, and it continues to be a significant concern for American children. Male and female toddlers and adolescent females are at greatest risk for iron-deficiency anemia; iron deficiency is reported in 14.4% of children aged 1 to 2 years and 9.3% of females aged 12 to 19 years.[9]

Biochemical Presentation

The biochemical presentation of iron-deficiency anemia varies depending on the cause and degree of iron deficiency. It is characterized by one or more of the following changes from age- and laboratory-specific norms:

- decreased hemoglobin (Hgb) and hematocrit (Hct)
- decreased mean cell volume (MCV)
- decreased transferrin saturation
- decreased serum ferritin
- increased total iron-binding capacity (TIBC)

Refer to Table 7.4 (pages 163 to 166) for normal laboratory values for iron.

Risk Factors

Risk factors for iron deficiency include the following:[5]

- prematurity or low birth weight
- exclusive breastfeeding beyond 4 months of age without supplemental iron
- low dietary iron intake during the first year as a result of weaning to whole milk or low-iron foods
- lead exposure
- low socioeconomic status (especially among people of Mexican American ethnicity)
- feeding problems, poor growth, and/or inadequate intake in children with special health care needs

Adolescent females are at risk due to menstrual losses and dietary patterns that may limit iron intake.[6] Both adolescent males and females who are involved in rigorous sports may also exhibit sports anemia. Children with chronic health conditions who require parenteral nutrition support are also at risk for iron deficiency, since iron is not routinely provided in parenteral nutrition.

Recommendations for supplementation to prevent development of iron deficiency or iron-deficiency anemia, including in exclusively breastfed infants between the ages of 4 and 6 months, can be found in Chapter 8.

Screening Guidelines

Screening for iron-deficiency anemia is routinely performed in both community and acute health care settings and involves evaluation of Hgb and Hct.

- **Infants:** The American Academy of Pediatrics recommends that all infants be screened for iron deficiency at approximately 12 months of age using a serum hemoglobin measurement.[6]

- **Preschool and school-age children:** Routine screening for anemia is not indicated for preschool and school-age children. However, annual screening should be performed for children between the ages of 2 and 5 years if they are at risk for iron deficiency because of special health needs, a low-iron diet (including diets that exclude meat or excessive milk intake), or environmental factors.[6] Screening for iron-deficiency anemia by finger stick is routinely done upon application of infants and children up to five for qualification to participate in the Special Supplemental Nutrition Program for Women, Infants, and Children.

- **Adolescents:** Adolescent should be screened for dietary practices that may put them at risk for iron-deficiency anemia during all routine physical exams and referred for testing.[6]

Other Anemias

Iron-deficiency anemia can be differentiated from other causes of anemia, including vitamin B-12 deficiency, folate deficiency, or chronic disease, by evaluation of hematologic indexes.

- In macrocytic anemia caused by vitamin B-12 or folate deficiency, Hgb and Hct are decreased; however, MCV and TIBC are increased, and transferrin saturation is normal.[10]

- In normocytic anemia of chronic disease, Hgb, Hct, TIBC, and transferrin saturation are decreased, while MCV is normal.[10]

Other Laboratory Values Relevant to Nutritional Status

Serum Electrolytes

Serum electrolytes, including sodium, potassium, and chloride, are used to evaluate hydration status and acid-base balance and may reflect renal function. Common chronic pediatric conditions, such as cystic fibrosis or renal disease, may also cause abnormal serum electrolyte levels.

Immune Markers

Immune markers of nutritional status include total lymphocyte count and delayed hypersensitivity to skin tests.

Medical Tests and Procedures

Box 7.1 describes selected medical tests and procedures used in pediatric nutrition assessment and their indications.[1,3,10-14]

BOX 7.1	Medical Tests and Procedures Used in Pediatric Nutrition Assessment[1,3,10-15]

Breath Hydrogen Test[11]

Measures hydrogen produced by bacterial fermentation of unabsorbed carbohydrate in the gastrointestinal tract

Possible indications:

Elevation of >20 ppm above baseline may indicate the following:

- carbohydrate (lactose, sucrose) malabsorption
- bacterial overgrowth (glucose)

Continued on next page

BOX 7.1   Medical Tests and Procedures Used in Pediatric Nutrition Assessment[1,3,10-15] (cont.)

Dual Energy X-Ray Absorptiometry

Measures bone density in the spine, hip, or forearm

Possible indications:

- Osteopenia due to prematurity, malabsorption, eating disorders, renal or hepatic disease
- Osteomalacia (rickets)
- Osteoporosis

Fecal Elastase-1 Test[12]

Measurement widely used to assess exocrine pancreatic function in children with cystic fibrosis; requires collection of stool sample

Normal values >500 mcg/g

Fecal Fat Test

Quantitative assessment of the percentage of dietary fat absorbed during a 72-hour period

Requires collection of all stools for 72 hours, combined with careful recording of dietary intake while consuming ≥25 g fat per day for infants and ≥100 g fat per day for children

Coefficient of absorption =

$$\frac{\text{Dietary Fat Consumed} - \text{Fecal Fat Excreted}}{\text{Dietary Fat Consumed}} \times 100$$

BOX 7.1   Medical Tests and Procedures Used in Pediatric Nutrition Assessment[1,3,10-15] (cont.)

Possible indications:

- Fat malabsorption may be due to diseases of gastrointestinal tract, including short bowel syndrome and cystic fibrosis
- In children and infants older than 6 months, fat loss in excess of 7% considered abnormal

Indirect Calorimetry[13]

Measures oxygen consumed and carbon dioxide produced to estimate Resting Energy Expenditure (REE)

Respiratory quotient (RQ) varies depending on the substrate being metabolized:

- RQ of fat = 0.7
- RQ of protein = 0.85
- RQ of carbohydrate = 1.0
- RQ for lipogenesis >1.0

Possible indications:

Measured Resting Energy Expenditures that vary greatly from predicted may indicate altered metabolic requirements (increased or decreased needs) or altered substrate utilization

Stool pH[14]

Measures the presence of fermented carbohydrate in stool

Possible indications:

pH <5.5 indicates carbohydrate malabsorption

Continued on next page

> ## BOX 7.1   Medical Tests and Procedures Used in Pediatric Nutrition Assessment[1,3,10-15] (cont.)
>
> ### Sweat Test[15]
> Measures sodium and chloride concentration in sweat
>
> **Possible indications:**
> High concentrations of chloride (>60 mmol/L) diagnostic of cystic fibrosis; levels between 30 and 59 mmol/L indicated possible cystic fibrosis and should be followed by additional testing
>
> ### Triene:Tetraene Ratio[16]
> Measures ratio of eicosatrienoic acid (20:3) to arachidonic acid (20:4) in blood
>
> **Possible indications:**
> Ratio is typically <0.1; elevated ratio >0.2 may indicate essential fatty acid deficiency

References

1.   Assessment of nutritional status. In: Kleinman RE, Greer FR, ed. *Pediatric Nutrition Handbook*. 7th ed. Elk Grove Village, IL: American Academy of Pediatrics; 2014:609-642.

2.   Ong C, Han WM, Wong JJM, Lee JH. Nutrition biomarkers and clinical outcomes in critically ill children: a critical appraisal of the literature. *Clin Nutr*. 2014;33:191-197.

3.   Loughrey CM, Young IS. Laboratory assessment of nutritional status. In: Duggan C, Watkins JB, Koletzko B, Walker WA, eds. *Nutrition in Pediatrics: Basic Science, Clinical Applications*. 5th ed. Shelton, CT: People's Medical Publishing House-USA; 2016.

4. Nutritional Disorders. In: *The Merck Manual Professional Version*. 2018. www.merckmanuals.com/professional /nutritional-disorders. Accessed September 10, 2018.

5. Baker RD, Greer FR, The Committee on Nutrition. Clinical report—diagnosis and prevention of iron deficiency and iron-deficient anemia in infants and young children (0-3 years of age). *Pediatrics*. 2010;126:1040-1050.

6. Iron. In: Kleinman RE, Greer FR, eds. *Pediatric Nutrition Handbook*. 7th ed. Elk Grove Village, IL: American Academy of Pediatrics; 2014:449-466.

7. Turner CB, Lin H, Flores G. Prevalence of vitamin D deficiency among overweight and obese US children. *Pediatrics*. 2013;131:e152-e161.

8. Golden NH, Abrams SA, Committee on Nutrition. Clinical report: optimizing bone health in children and adolescents. *Pediatrics*. 2014;134:e1229-e1243.

9. Cogswell ME, Looker AC, Pfeiffer CM, et al. Assessment of iron deficiency in US preschool children and nonpregnant females of childbearing age: National Health and Nutrition Examination Survey 2003-2006. *Am J Clin Nutr*. 2009;89:1334-1342.

10. Nevin-Folino N, LeBeouf-Aufdenkampe R. Laboratory assessment. In: Baker SS, Baker RD, Davis AM, eds. *Pediatric Nutrition Support*. Sudbury, MA: Jones and Bartlett; 2007:83-95.

11. Chronic diarrheal disease. In: Kleinman RE, Greer FR, eds. *Pediatric Nutrition Handbook*. 7th ed. Elk Grove Village, IL: American Academy of Pediatrics; 2014:701-716.

12. Wali PD, Loveridge-Lenza B, He Z, Horvath K. Comparison of fecal elastase-1 and pancreatic function testing in children. *J Pediatr Gastroint Nutr*. 2012;54:277-280.

13. Energy. In: Kleinman RE, Greer FR, eds. *Pediatric Nutrition Handbook*. 7th ed. Elk Grove Village, IL: American Academy of Pediatrics; 2014:359-368.

14. Carbohydrates and dietary fiber. In: Kleinman RE, Greer FR, eds. *Pediatric Nutrition Handbook*. 7th ed. Elk Grove Village, IL: American Academy of Pediatrics; 2014:387-406.

15. Farrell PM, Rosenstein BJ, White TB, et al. Guidelines for diagnosis of cystic fibrosis in newborns through older adults: Cystic Fibrosis Foundation Consensus Report. *J Pediatr*. 2008;153:S4-S14.

16. Fats and fatty acids. In: Kleinman RE, Greer FR, eds. *Pediatric Nutrition Handbook*. 7th ed. Elk Grove Village, IL: American Academy of Pediatrics; 2014:407-434.

CHAPTER 8

Energy and Nutrient Requirements

Because of their increased needs for growth and development, infants, children, and adolescents have nutrient requirements proportionately higher per kilogram of body mass than those of adults. This chapter provides comparative nutritional standards for use in the assessment of pediatric patients/clients, methods of estimating energy needs, and nutrients of particular concern in the pediatric population.

Dietary Reference Intakes

Estimated nutrient intakes can be described in terms of the Dietary Reference Intakes (DRIs), a set of nutrient-based reference values developed by the Institute of Medicine's Food and Nutrition Board, to be used for planning and assessing diets.[1] Practitioners should monitor and use the most recent DRI values published.

Definitions

The DRIs are defined as follows:[1]

- **Estimated Average Requirement (EAR):** the median usual intake that is estimated to meet the requirement of half the healthy population for age and gender (At this level of intake, half the individuals will have their nutrient needs met.)

- **Recommended Dietary Allowance (RDA):** the level sufficient to meet the nutrient requirement of nearly all (97% to 98%) healthy individuals

- **Adequate Intake (AI):** an approximation of intake by a group of healthy individuals maintaining a defined nutritional status

- **Tolerable Upper Intake Level (UL):** the highest level of ongoing daily intake of a nutrient that is estimated to pose no risk in almost all individuals

- **Estimated Energy Requirement (EER):** the dietary energy intake of children, adolescents, and pregnant or lactating adolescents for a given age, gender, and level of physical activity that is predicted to maintain energy balance and to allow for appropriate tissue deposition

Where adequate information exists, each nutrient has either an EAR and RDA or an AI. In addition, many nutrients have a UL.

Dietary Reference Intakes for Infants

Because there is insufficient evidence for nutrient requirements in infancy, the EAR and RDA have been established only for protein and iron for infants between 7 and 12 months; all other nutrients have been assigned an AI. DRIs have not yet been established for preterm infants.

- For infants in the first 6 months of life, the AI is generally based on the daily mean intake provided by breastmilk to an exclusively breastfed, full-term baby who is growing appropriately.

- For infants aged 7 to 12 months, the AI is based on usual intake of breastmilk combined with the usual intake of complementary foods.

Interpretation of Individual Intakes versus Dietary Reference Intakes

When assessing an individual's nutrient intake, it may be useful to consider that typical intakes below the EAR very likely need to be improved, and those between the EAR and RDA probably need to be improved. Although it can be assumed that typical intakes that equal or exceed the AI are adequate, it is difficult to interpret typical intakes below the AI. Finally, if typical intake exceeds the UL, it may pose a risk to some healthy individuals.[1]

Because the DRIs are based on healthy children, they should be viewed as a starting point from which to consider modification of nutrient recommendations for children with acute or chronic illnesses. For example, individual differences in nutrient requirements, metabolic stress, physical inactivity, and illnesses and medications that affect absorption or excretion of nutrients can all have an impact on nutrient needs.

Clinical, biochemical, and functional nutritional status should be considered along with dietary intake in determining individual nutrient needs. In addition, the DRIs may be used to estimate nutrient requirements for oral/enteral intake, but they are *not* appropriate for calculating requirements for parenteral nutrition. See Tables 8.1 to 8.4 (pages 181 to 192) for Dietary Reference Intakes by gender and age.

TABLE 8.1   Dietary Reference Intakes, Males and Females Aged 0 to 8 Years[2,3]

Nutrient	0–6 mo	6–12 mo	1–3 y	4–8 y
Water (L/d)	0.7[a]	0.8[a]	1.3[a]	1.7[a]
Carbohydrates (g/d)	60[a]	95[a]	130 (45%–65% of kcal)	130 (45%–65% of kcal)
Fiber (g/d)	Not determined	Not determined	19[a]	25[a]
Fat (g/d)	31[a]	30[a]	Not determined (30%–40% of kcal)	Not determined (25%–35% of kcal)
Linoleic acid (g/d)	4.4[a]	4.6[a]	7[a] (5%–10% of kcal)	10[a] (5%–10% of kcal)
α-Linolenic acid (g/d)	0.5[a]	0.5[a]	0.7[a] (0.6%–1.2% of kcal)	0.9[a] (0.6%–1.2% of kcal)
Protein (g/d)	9.1[a]	11.0	13 (5%–20% of kcal)	19 (10%–30% of kcal)
Vitamin A (µg/d)	400[a]	500[a]	300	400
Vitamin C (mg/d)	40[a]	50[a]	15	25
Vitamin D (µg/d)	10[a]	10[a]	15	15
Vitamin E (mg/d)	4[a]	5[a]	6	7

Continued on next page

TABLE 8.1 Dietary Reference Intakes, Males and Females Aged 0 to 8 Years[2,3] (cont.)				
Nutrient	0–6 mo	6–12 mo	1–3 y	4–8 y
Vitamin K (μg/d)	2.0[a]	2.5[a]	30[a]	55[a]
Thiamin (mg/d)	0.2[a]	0.3[a]	0.5	0.6
Riboflavin (mg/d)	0.3[a]	0.4[a]	0.5	0.6
Niacin (mg/d)	2[a]	4[a]	6	8
Vitamin B-6 (mg/d)	0.1[a]	0.3[a]	0.5	0.6
Folate (μg/d)	65[a]	80[a]	150	200
Vitamin B-12 (μg/d)	0.4[a]	0.5[a]	0.9	1.2
Pantothenic acid (mg/d)	1.7[a]	1.8[a]	2[a]	3[a]
Biotin (μg/d)	5[a]	6[a]	8[a]	12[a]
Choline (mg/d)	125[a]	150[a]	200[a]	250[a]
Calcium (mg/d)	200[a]	260[a]	700	1,000
Chromium (μg/d)	0.2[a]	5.5[a]	11[a]	15[a]
Copper (μg/d)	200[a]	220[a]	340	440
Fluoride (mg/d)	0.01[a]	0.5[a]	0.7[a]	1[a]

Iodine (µg/d)	110[a]	130[a]	90	90
Iron (mg/d)	0.27[a]	11	7	10
Magnesium (mg/d)	30[a]	75[a]	80	130
Manganese (mg/d)	0.003[a]	0.6[a]	1.2[a]	1.5[a]
Molybdenum (µg/d)	2[a]	3[a]	17	22
Phosphorus (mg/d)	100[a]	275[a]	460	500
Selenium (µg/d)	15[a]	20[a]	20	30
Zinc (mg/d)	2[a]	3	3	5
Potassium (g/d)	0.4[a]	0.7[a]	3.0[a]	3.8[a]
Sodium (g/d)	0.12[a]	0.37	1.0[a]	1.2[a]
Chloride (g/d)	0.18[a]	0.57[a]	1.5[a]	1.9[a]

[a] Adequate intake

TABLE 8.2 Dietary Reference Intakes, Males Aged 9 to 30 Years[2,3]			
Nutrient	9–13 y	14–18 y	19–30 y
Water (L/d)	2.4[a]	3.3[a]	3.7[a]
Carbohydrates (g/d)	130 (45%–65% of kcal)	130 (45%–65% of kcal)	130 (45%–65% of kcal)
Fiber (g/d)	31[a]	38[a]	38[a]
Fat (g/d)	Not determined (25%–35% of kcal)	Not determined (255%–35% of kcal)	Not determined (20%–35% of kcal)
Linoleic acid (g/d)	12[a] (5%–10% of kcal)	16[a] (5%–10% of kcal)	17[a] (5%–10% of kcal)
α-Linolenic acid (g/d)	1.2[a] (0.6%–1.2% of kcal)	1.6[a] (0.6%–1.2% of kcal)	1.6[a] (0.6%–1.2% of kcal)
Protein (g/d)	34 (10%–30% of kcal)	52 (10%–30% of kcal)	56 (10%–35% of kcal)
Vitamin A (μg/d)	600	900	900
Vitamin C (mg/d)	45	75	90
Vitamin D (μg/d)	15	15	15
Vitamin E (mg/d)	11	15	15
Vitamin K (μg/d)	60[a]	75[a]	120[a]

Thiamin (mg/d)	0.9	1.2	1.2
Riboflavin (mg/d)	0.9	1.3	1.3
Niacin (mg/d)	12	16	16
Vitamin B-6 (mg/d)	1.0	1.3	1.3
Folate (µg/d)	300	400	400
Vitamin B-12 (µg/d)	1.8	2.4	2.4
Pantothenic acid (mg/d)	4[a]	5[a]	5[a]
Biotin (µg/d)	20[a]	25[a]	30[a]
Choline (mg/d)	375[a]	550[a]	550[a]
Calcium (mg/d)	1,300	1,300	1,000
Chromium (µg/d)	25[a]	35[a]	35[a]
Copper (µg/d)	700	890	900
Fluoride (mg/d)	2[a]	3[a]	4[a]
Iodine (µg/d)	120	150	150
Iron (mg/d)	8	11	8
Magnesium (mg/d)	240	410	400
Manganese (mg/d)	1.9[a]	2.2[a]	2.3[a]

Continued on next page

Energy and
Nutrients

TABLE 8.2   Dietary Reference Intakes, Males Aged 9 to 30 Years[2,3] (cont.)

Nutrient	9–13 y	14–18 y	19–30 y
Molybdenum (μg/d)	34	43	45
Phosphorus (mg/d)	1,250	1,250	700
Selenium (μg/d)	40	55	55
Zinc (mg/d)	8	11	11
Potassium (g/d)	4.5[a]	4.7[a]	4.7[a]
Sodium (g/d)	1.5[a]	1.5[a]	1.5[a]
Chloride (g/d)	2.3[a]	2.3[a]	2.3[a]

[a] Adequate intake

TABLE 8.3 Dietary Reference Intakes, Females Aged 9 to 30 Years[2,3]

Nutrient	9–13 y	14–18 y	19–30 y
Water (L/d)	2.1[a]	2.3[a]	2.7[a]
Carbohydrates (g/d)	130 (45%–65% of kcal)	130 (45%–65% of kcal)	130 (45%–65% of kcal)
Fiber (g/d)	26[a]	26[a]	25[a]
Fat (g/d)	Not determined (25%–35% of kcal)	Not determined (25%–35% of kcal)	Not determined (20%–35% of kcal)
Linoleic acid (g/d)	10[a] (5%–10% of kcal)	11[a] (5%–10% of kcal)	12[a] (5%–10% of kcal)
α-Linolenic acid (g/d)	1.0[a] (0.6%–1.2% of kcal)	1.1[a] (0.6%–1.2% of kcal)	1.1[a] (0.6%–1.2% of kcal)
Protein (g/d)	34 (10%–30% of kcal)	46 (10%–30% of kcal)	46 (10%–35% of kcal)
Vitamin A (μg/d)	600	700	700
Vitamin C (mg/d)	45	65	75
Vitamin D (μg/d)	15	15	15
Vitamin E (mg/d)	11	15	15

Continued on next page

TABLE 8.3 Dietary Reference Intakes, Females Aged 9 to 30 Years[2,3] (cont.)

Nutrient	9–13 y	14–18 y	19–30 y
Vitamin K (μg/d)	60[a]	75[a]	90[a]
Thiamin (mg/d)	0.9	1.0	1.1
Riboflavin (mg/d)	0.9	1.0	1.1
Niacin (mg/d)	12	14	14
Vitamin B-6 (mg/d)	1.0	1.2	1.3
Folate (μg/d)	300	400	400
Vitamin B-12 (μg/d)	1.8	2.4	2.4
Pantothenic acid (mg/d)	4[a]	5[a]	5[a]
Biotin (μg/d)	20[a]	25[a]	30[a]
Choline (mg/d)	375[a]	400[a]	425[a]
Calcium (mg/d)	1,300	1,300	1,000
Chromium (μg/d)	21[a]	24[a]	25[a]
Copper (μg/d)	700	890	900
Fluoride (mg/d)	2[a]	3[a]	3[a]
Iodine (μg/d)	120	150	150
Iron (mg/d)	8	15	18

Magnesium (mg/d)	240	360	310
Manganese (mg/d)	1.6[a]	1.6[a]	1.8[a]
Molybdenum (μg/d)	34	43	45
Phosphorus (mg/d)	1,250	1,250	700
Selenium (μg/d)	40	55	55
Zinc (mg/d)	8	9	8
Potassium (g/d)	4.5[a]	4.7[a]	4.7[a]
Sodium (g/d)	1.5[a]	1.5[a]	1.5[a]
Chloride (g/d)	2.3[a]	2.3[a]	2.3[a]

[a] Adequate intake

TABLE 8.4 Dietary Reference Intakes, Pregnant and Lactating Females Aged 14 to 30 Years[2,3]

Nutrient	Pregnancy 14–18 y	Pregnancy 19–30 y	Lactation 14–18 y	Lactation 19–30 y
Water (L/d)	3.0[a]	3.0[a]	3.8[a]	3.8[a]
Carbohydrates (g/d)	175 (45%–65% of kcal)	175 (45%–65% of kcal)	210 (45%–65% of kcal)	210 (45%–65% of kcal)
Fiber (g/d)	28[a]	28[a]	29[a]	29[a]
Fat (g/d)	Not determined (25%–35% of kcal)	Not determined (20%–35% of kcal)	Not determined (25%–35% of kcal)	Not determined (20%–35% of kcal)
Linoleic acid (g/d)	13[a] (5%–10% of kcal)	13[a] (5%–10% of kcal)	13[a] (5%–10% of kcal)	13[a] (5%–10% of kcal)
α-Linolenic acid (g/d)	1.4[a] (0.6%–1.2% of kcal)	1.4[a] (0.6%–1.2% of kcal)	1.3[a] (0.6%–1.2% of kcal)	1.3[a] (0.6%–1.2% of kcal)
Protein (g/d)	71 (10%–30% of kcal)	71 (10%–35% of kcal)	71 (10%–30% of kcal)	71 (10%–35% of kcal)

Vitamin A (µg/d)	750	770	1,200	1,300
Vitamin C (mg/d)	80	85	115	120
Vitamin D (µg/d)	15	15	15	15
Vitamin E (mg/d)	15	15	19	19
Vitamin K (µg/d)	75[a]	90[a]	75[a]	90[a]
Thiamin (mg/d)	1.4	1.4	1.4	1.4
Riboflavin (mg/d)	1.4	1.4	1.6	1.6
Niacin (mg/d)	18	18	17	17
Vitamin B-6 (mg/d)	1.9	1.9	2.0	2.0
Folate (µg/d)	600	600	500	500
Vitamin B-12 (µg/d)	2.6	2.6	2.8	2.8
Pantothenic acid (mg/d)	6[a]	6[a]	7[a]	7[a]
Biotin (µg/d)	30[a]	30[a]	35[a]	35[a]
Choline (mg/d)	450[a]	450[a]	550[a]	550[a]
Calcium (mg/d)	1,300	1,000	1,300	1,000
Chromium (µg/d)	29[a]	30[a]	44[a]	45[a]
Copper (µg/d)	1,000	1,000	1,300	1,300

Continued on next page

Energy and
Nutrients

Energy and
Nutrients

TABLE 8.4   Dietary Reference Intakes, Pregnant and Lactating Females Aged 14 to 30 Years[2,3] (cont.)

Nutrient	Pregnancy 14–18 y	Pregnancy 19–30 y	Lactation 14–18 y	Lactation 19–30 y
Fluoride (mg/d)	3[a]	3[a]	3[a]	3[a]
Iodine (μg/d)	220	220	290	290
Iron (mg/d)	27	27	10	9
Magnesium (mg/d)	400	350	360	310
Manganese (mg/d)	2.0[a]	2.0[a]	2.6[a]	2.6[a]
Molybdenum (μg/d)	50	50	50	50
Phosphorus (mg/d)	1,250	700	1,250	700
Selenium (μg/d)	60	60	70	70
Zinc (mg/d)	12	11	13	12
Potassium (g/d)	4.7[a]	4.7[a]	5.1[a]	5.1[a]
Sodium (g/d)	1.5[a]	1.5[a]	1.5[a]	1.5[a]
Chloride (g/d)	2.3[a]	2.3[a]	2.3[a]	2.3[a]

[a] Adequate intake

Energy Requirements

Energy requirements can be estimated with predictive equations or measured by indirect calorimetry. The specific method or equation chosen depends on the setting, availability of data, and the child's clinical status. It is important to emphasize that estimates of energy requirements using measured indirect calorimetry or predictive equations provide only a starting point. Each child's actual weight gain and growth should be closely monitored and energy goals adjusted appropriately.

Indirect Calorimetry

Indirect calorimetry is the most accurate method for determining individual energy requirements. However, because access to equipment is limited and testing may be expensive or impractical, its use is limited.

Estimated Energy Requirements

For well infants, children, and adolescents and those in ambulatory settings, the EER can be calculated with appropriate DRI prediction equations derived from daily energy expenditure as measured by the doubly labeled water technique. The EER for infants and young children up to 35 months is based on needs for total energy expenditure (TEE) and needs for energy deposition for growth. See Table 8.5 (page 194) for age-specific equations.[3]

TABLE 8.5	Estimated Energy Requirements for Infants and Young Children[3]
Age, mo	Estimated Energy Requirements, kcal/d
0–3	(89 × weight of infant [kg]) + 75
4–6	(89 × weight of infant [kg]) – 44
7–12	(89 × weight of infant [kg]) – 78
13–36	(89 × weight of child [kg]) – 80

For children aged 3 years and older and for adolescents, the EER equations include additional factors to account for height and physical activity. See Tables 8.6 and 8.7 (pages 195 and 196) for the appropriate formulas and physical activity factors.[3] As noted in Chapter 5, Table 5.3 (pages 135 to 137) provides very broad estimated calorie needs of healthy children based on reference (average) heights and reference (healthy) weights for age and sex; however, they do not account for individual differences for children who differ from the norm.

NOTE: Users must follow standard mathematical rules for order of operations (parentheses, exponents, multiplication or division, and addition or subtraction).

Sample calculation for a boy, aged 4 years, who is active, weighing 16.0 kg and measuring 103 cm tall:

$$\begin{aligned}
\text{EER} &= 108.5 - (61.9 \times 4) + 1.26 \times \{(26.7 \times 16.0) \\
&\quad + (903 \times 103)\} \\
&= 108.5 - (247.6) + 1.26 \times \{(427.2) + (800)\} \\
&= 108.5 - 247.6 + (1.26 \times 1{,}227.2) \\
&= 108.5 - 247.6 + 1{,}546.3 \\
&= 1{,}407.2 \text{ kcal/day}
\end{aligned}$$

TABLE 8.6 Estimated Energy Requirements for Boys and Girls Aged 3 to 18 Years[3]

Age, y	Estimated Energy Requirements, kcal/d
3–8	**Boys:** 108.5 – (61.9 × age [y]) + PA[a] × {(26.7 × weight [kg]) + (903 × height [m])}
	Girls: 155.3 – (30.8 × age [y]) + PA × {(10.0 × weight [kg]) + (934 × height [m])}
9–18	**Boys:** 113.5 – (61.9 × age [y]) + PA ×{(26.7 × weight [kg]) + (903 × height [m])}
	Girls: 160.3 – (30.8 × age [y]) + PA × {(10.0 × weight [kg])+ (934 × height [m])}

[a] PA, physical activity coefficient (see Table 8.7)

TABLE 8.7	**Physical Activity Coefficients for Normal-Weight Boys and Girls Aged 3 to 18 Years[3]**		
Physical activity level[a]	**Activity Required**	**Physical Activity Coefficient**	
		Boys	**Girls**
Sedentary	Lying awake; sitting	1.00	1.00
Low active	Activity equivalent to walking ~120 min at 2.5 mph	1.13	1.16
Active	Activity equivalent to walking ~230 min at 2.5 mph	1.26	1.31
Very active	Activity equivalent to walking ~400 min at 2.5 mph	1.42	1.56

[a] Physical activity level (PAL) is defined as the ratio of total energy expenditure to basal energy expenditure. PAL is determined from assessment of the amount of time the child or adolescent spends in moderate and vigorous play and work

Estimates for Children with Chronic Health Conditions

Energy requirements may be altered by either acute or chronic illness. See Box 8.1 for methods used to estimate energy requirements for children with chronic health conditions.[4] Although these methods may be useful in estimating requirements, they should be viewed as estimates only. In practice, it is often useful to calculate estimated needs by several different methods, compare results, and apply clinical judgment.

BOX 8.1   Alternative Methods of Estimating Daily Energy Requirements Based on Health Condition[6,12]

Down Syndrome

14.3 kcal/cm for girls aged 5–11 y

16.1 kcal/cm for boys aged 5–11 y

Spina Bifida

Children older than 8 y who are minimally active:

- To maintain weight: 9–11 kcal/cm, or 50% fewer kcal than recommended for a child of the same age without the condition
- To promote weight loss: 7 kcal/cm

Prader-Willi Syndrome

For all children and adolescents:

- 10–11 kcal/cm to maintain growth within a growth channel
- 8.5 kcal/cm for slow weight loss and support linear growth

Cerebral Palsy

Ambulatory, ages 5–12 y: 13.9 kcal/cm

Nonambulatory, ages 5–12 y: 11.1 kcal/cm

Cerebral palsy with severely restricted activity: 10 kcal/cm

Cerebral palsy with mild-to-moderate activity: 15 kcal/cm

Continued on next page

BOX 8.1   Alternative Methods of Estimating Daily Energy Requirements Based on Health Condition[7,11] (cont.)

Failure to Thrive

Energy requirement will depend on etiology or medical condition, but start with Estimated Energy Requirement (EER) calculations using ideal body weight for height-age and EER for height-age. *Height-age* is defined as age at which current height or length would fall at the 50th percentile on the height-for-age or length-for-age growth chart (see Chapter 1). *Ideal body weight for height-age* is defined as weight at the 50th percentile for height-age. *Example:* A female aged 9 months with weight of 6.4 kg and length of 66 cm (height-age = 6 mo). Ideal body weight for a female aged 6 months is 7.3 kg.

EER (kcal/d) = (89 × Weight [kg] − 100) + 56
            = (89 × 7.3 − 100) + 56 = 606

To calculate estimated catch-up growth needs, use the following formula:

Energy needs (kcal/d) = (EER for Age × Ideal Weight for
                        Height [kg])/Actual Weight (kg)

Cystic Fibrosis

Calculate ideal weight based on height, using the pediatric growth chart. Multiply by the child's EER for age. Multiply by a factor of 1.3 to 1.5 (depending on the severity of the disease) to compensate for increased energy demands.

Estimates for Children with Acute Illnesses

For acutely ill children, equations that predict resting energy expenditure (REE) may be used. The World Health Organization[6] and Schofield[7] have developed predictive equations that are often used to calculate REEs for hospitalized pediatric patients (see Tables 8.8 and 8.9 on pages 199 and 120). The REE may then be multiplied by stress factors to account for altered energy requirements due to specific clinical conditions (see Table 8.10, page 200).[6,9] It is important, however, to avoid overfeeding the critically ill child because pulmonary and hepatic complications may occur. Feedings should be advanced slowly as tolerated.

TABLE 8.8	World Health Organization Equations for Estimating Resting Energy Expenditures[6]
Age, y	Resting Energy Expenditures, kcal/d
0–3	Males: (60.9 × weight [kg]) – 54 Females: (61.0 × weight [kg]) – 51
3–10	Males: (22.7 × weight [kg]) + 495 Females: (22.5 × weight [kg]) + 499
10–18	Males: (17.5 × weight [kg]) + 651 Females: (12.2 × weight [kg]) + 746

TABLE 8.9 Schofield Equations for Estimating Resting Energy Expenditures[7]

Age, y	Resting Energy Expenditures, kcal/d
0–3	Males: (0.167 × weight [kg]) + (15.174 × height [cm]) − 617.6 Females: (16.252 × weight [kg]) + (10.232 × height [cm]) − 413.5
3–10	Males: (19.59 × weight [kg]) + (1.303 × height [cm]) + 414.9 Females: (16.969 × weight [kg]) + (1.618 × height [cm]) + 371.2
10–18	Males: (16.25 × weight [kg]) + (1.372 × height [cm]) − 515.5 Females: (8.365 × weight [kg]) + (4.65 × height [cm]) + 200
>18	Males: (15.057 × weight [kg]) + (1.0004 × height [cm]) + 705.8 Females: (13.623 × weight [kg]) + (23.8 × height [cm]) + 98.2

TABLE 8.10 Stress Factors and Effects on Energy Requirements[a,8,9]

Type of Stress	Multiply Resting Energy Expenditures By
Starvation	0.70–0.85
Surgery	1.05–1.5
Sepsis	1.2–1.6
Closed head injury	1.3
Trauma	1.1–1.8
Growth failure	1.5–2.0
Burn	1.5–2.5

[a] See Tables 8.8 and 8.9 for REE equations.

Estimates for Overweight/Obese Children

Separate predictive equations for energy requirements to maintain weight have been developed for children whose body mass indexes are greater than the 95th percentile for age and gender. See Tables 8.11 and 8.12.[3,10]

TABLE 8.11 Total Energy Expenditure for Weight Maintenance in Obese[a] Boys and Girls Aged 3 to 18 Years[3]

Gender	Total Energy Expenditure, kcal/d
Boys	$-114 - (50.9 \times \text{age [y]}) + PA \times \{(19.5 \times \text{weight [kg]}) + (1161.4 \times \text{height [m]})\}$
Girls	$389 - (41.2 \times \text{age [y]}) + PA \times \{(15.0 \times \text{weight [kg]}) + (701.6 \times \text{height [m]})\}$

[a] Obesity is defined as body mass index >95th percentile for age and gender

TABLE 8.12 Physical Activity Coefficients for Obese[a] Boys and Girls Aged 3 to 18 Years[3]

Physical Activity Level[b]	Physical Activity Coefficient	
	Boys	Girls
Sedentary	1.00	1.00
Low active	1.12	1.18
Active	1.24	1.35
Very active	1.45	1.60

[a] Obesity is defined as body mass index >95th percentile for age and sex.
[b] Physical activity level (PAL) is defined as the ratio of total energy expenditure to basal energy expenditure.[3] PAL is determined from assessment of the amount of time the child or adolescent spends in moderate and vigorous play and work

Equations to predict the basal metabolic rate (BMR) in obese children and adolescents have been published (see Table 8.13, page 202).[11] Since these calculations predict only resting energy needs, results obtained using these equations should be adjusted for physical activity to determine total energy needs. As with normal-weight children, other predictive equations may be used to estimate energy needs for hospitalized overweight children (see Tables 8.8 and 8.9 on pages 199 and 200).

TABLE 8.13	Basal Metabolic Rate Prediction Equations for Obese Children and Adolescents, Aged 7 to 18 Years Basal Metabolic Rate[11]
Males	Basal Metabolic Rate = 238.85 {(weight [kg] × 0.044) + (height [cm] × 0.02836) − (pubertal stage[a] × 0.148) + 0.23)}
Females	Basal Metabolic Rate = 238.85 {(weight [kg] × 0.044) + (height [cm] × 0.02836) − (pubertal stage[a] × 0.148) − 0.551}

[a] Pubertal stage in values from 1 to 5

Estimates for Pregnant and Lactating Adolescents

EER equations are provided for pregnancy and lactation during adolescence (see Table 8.14).[3]

TABLE 8.14	Estimated Energy Requirements for Pregnant and Lactating Adolescents[3]	
	Stage	**Energy Needs (kcal/d)**
PregRev 3	First trimester	Estimated Energy Requirements (EER) for age[a] + 0
	Second trimester	EER for age[a] + 340
	Third trimester	EER for age[a] + 452
Lactation	First 6 mo	EER for age[a] + 330
	Second 6 mo	EER for age[a] + 400

[a] For girls 14 to 18 years, use adolescent Estimated Energy Requirements; for females 19 years or older, use adult Estimated Energy Requirements.

Nutrient Requirements of Special Concern in Pediatrics

The Academy of Nutrition and Dietetics, the American Academy of Pediatrics (AAP), and the American Medical Association (AMA) recommend that foods serve as the primary source of nutrients.[12,13] However, the AAP recognizes certain groups at nutritional risk who may benefit from supplementation (see Box 8.2, page 204).[13] Care must be taken to avoid excess intakes of some nutrients, especially those commonly found in supplements and in fortified foods, such as vitamin A, zinc, and folate.[14] In addition, the following sections outline specific risks for nutrient inadequacy and appropriate supplementation.

See Chapter 7 for guidance on using biochemical data to evaluate nutrient adequacy.

> ### BOX 8.2   Nutritional Risks in Children That May Benefit from Supplementation[13]
>
> - Anorexia, inadequate appetite, or following a fad diet
> - Chronic disease (eg, cystic fibrosis, inflammatory bowel disease, malabsorption syndromes, or hepatic disease)
> - Food insecurity or history of neglect or abuse
> - Participation in a dietary program for obesity management
> - Consumption of a vegetarian diet without adequate dairy products
> - Malnutrition
> - Use of medications with known nutrition implications
> - Multiple severe food allergies limiting food variety and nutrient density
> - History of extreme prematurity
> - Hypocaloric tube feeding regimen for children with low energy needs

Vitamin K

Because of the low levels of vitamin K in human milk, the inadequate production of vitamin K from bacteria in the gastrointestinal tract in early infancy, and the risk of fatal brain hemorrhage due to vitamin K deficiency, the AAP recommends that all infants receive an intramuscular injection of vitamin K at birth, regardless of the mother's plans to breast- or bottle-feed.[15] A systematic review of the literature affirmed this recommendation and identified the need for studies to compare the efficacy of a single intramuscular dose at birth to multiple oral doses over the first month of life.[16]

Vitamin D

Cases of vitamin D deficiency rickets in breastfed infants in the 1990s to 2000s,[17] and concerns for the harmful effects of early sun exposure have resulted in the AAP recommendation that all infants have a minimum daily intake of 400 IU of supplemental vitamin D beginning soon after birth.[18-20] Breastfed infants should receive a supplement of 400 IU of vitamin D beginning in the first few days of life; alternatively, lactating mothers may supplement their diet with 6,000 to 6,400 IU per day of vitamin D to increase the vitamin D content of their breastmilk.[20-22] This requirement may also be met with infant formula for infants who are consuming at least 1 liter (~1 quart) of standard infant formula or cow's milk (if less than 12 months of age) daily. Beginning at 1 year of age, children and adolescents should receive 600 IU of vitamin D daily.[3,20] It should also be noted that children who are obese or are taking certain medications, including glucocorticoids, antifungals, anticonvulsants, or antiretrovirals, may have higher vitamin D requirements.[20] Sufficiency of intake or supplementation and screening of children at risk should be evaluated by measuring serum 25-hydroxyvitamin D.

In spite of these recommendations, research indicates that only 20% to 37% of formula-fed infants, 9% to 14% of mixed-fed infants, and 5% to 13% of infants who were exclusively fed breastmilk met the recommended levels of intake.[23,24] Dietary intake data of US toddlers aged 12 to 23 months shows that 74% are consuming less than the EAR.[24] Vitamin D insufficiency and deficiency have been reported to occur in as many as 69% to 97% of pregnant women, with greater incidence among women early in pregnancy and those who are African American.[25,26] These suboptimal levels directly impact the developing fetus, which depends entirely on maternal stores. Attention should be given to ensuring AI during pregnancy and lactation to ensure sufficient vitamin D in the infant.

Vitamin D deficiency rickets has been reported in toddlers on a vegan (strict vegetarian) diet or breastfed by mothers on vegan diets.[27] Some milk alternatives used for toddlers and older children on vegan diets, such as soy or rice milks, contain inadequate vitamin D to prevent deficiency, especially in darkly pigmented children; fortified soy and rice milks should be carefully evaluated for nutrient sufficiency.

Assuming minimal sun exposure, the recommended intake of vitamin D for all children aged 12 months and older is 600 IU per day.[19] Guidelines for screening for vitamin D deficiency are discussed in Chapter 7.

Iron

Infants

Full-term infants have adequate iron stores to last until 4 to 6 months of age; preterm and low-birth-weight infants may deplete their iron stores as early as 2 to 3 months of age. The AAP recommends that full-term infants receive approximately 1 mg/kg of iron daily starting at 4 months of age.[28,29] Preterm infants should receive 2 mg/kg of iron daily starting at 1 month of age.[29]

Some research indicates that better visual acuity and higher motor test scores at age 12 months were achieved when breastfed infants received supplemental iron between 1 and 6 months of age.[30] Although studies have demonstrated that earlier administration of supplemental iron is safe,[31] it is still not clear whether it provides measurable benefits.[32]

All breastfed infants younger than 12 months should receive only iron-fortified infant formula as a supplement to breastmilk or when weaning from the breast. Formula-fed infants should receive only iron-fortified formula. Cow, goat, or soy milk should not be offered to infants before 1 year of age. Although the amount of iron in infant formulas is adequate to meet the needs of full-term infants, preterm infants who are formula fed with standard infant formula may need additional supplemental iron to meet the 2 mg/kg/day recommendation.

Infants between 6 and 12 months of age should consume 11 mg iron per day.[29] For older infants, the addition of approximately 1 mg/kg of iron per day can be accomplished by the introduction of two servings a day of iron-fortified infant cereal (½ oz per serving), meats, or a combination of cereal and meats.

Children Aged 1 to 5 Years

Children between the ages of 1 and 5 years are at greatest risk for iron deficiency. According to the most recent data published by the Centers for Disease Control and Prevention from the National Health and Nutrition Examination Survey (NHANES), approximately 9% of children aged 1 to 5 years are iron deficient, as measured by a serum ferritin concentration below the minimum acceptable level (<12 ng/mL).[33]

The AAP recommends that *all* children be screened for iron deficiency at approximately 12 months of age using hemoglobin (Hgb) concentration, as well as assessment of risk factors (see Chapter 7 for list of risk factors to assess).[28]

Children whose Hgb concentration on screening is less than 11.0 mg/dL should have further evaluation for iron-deficiency anemia, including measurement of *both* serum ferritin *and* C-reactive protein *or* of reticulocyte Hgb. Because ferritin is an acute-phase reactant, its measurement must be combined with measurement of C-reactive protein to rule out inflammation; a child whose Hgb concentration on screening is between 10.0 and 11.0 mg/dL should be closely monitored.[28] *See* Chapter 7 for additional information on assessment of laboratory values for iron.

Adolescents

Adolescent males are at risk for iron-deficiency anemia during their peak growth spurt, when iron stores may not be adequate for the demand of rapid growth; they should be screened for anemia as part of a routine physical exam during the period of peak growth during adolescence.[29]

Adolescent females are at risk for iron-deficiency anemia due to menstrual blood losses. Data from the NHANES indicate that 9.3% of nonpregnant females between 12 and 19 years of age are iron deficient.[34] Adolescent females should be screened for anemia during all routine physical exams.[29]

Fluoride

Fluoride supplementation has been demonstrated to be beneficial in reducing the incidence of early childhood caries and has significantly improved the oral health of the nation.[35] A child's need for fluoride supplementation depends on the total amount of fluoride available from all sources, including infant formula, tap and bottled water, and commercial and home-prepared foods. In 2015, the United States Health and Human Services Public Health Service released an updated recommendation that the optimal fluoride concentration in community water systems is 0.7 mg/L.[36] Information on fluoridation of public water supplies can be found on the Centers for Disease Control and Prevention website (www.cdc.gov /fluoridation/index.html).

Comprehensive reviews of published clinical trials have confirmed the efficacy of recommendations on the use of dietary fluoride supplements.[37] See Table 8.15 for the clinical recommendations for the use of dietary fluoride supplements from birth to 16 years of age.[38] Dietary fluoride supplements are not recommended for children at low risk of developing dental caries; other sources of fluoride should be considered. Dietary fluoride supplements, when prescribed, should be taken daily.

TABLE 8.15	Clinical Recommendations for the Use of Dietary Fluoride Supplements[38]		
	Level of Fluoride Ion in Drinking Water (ppm)[a]		
Age	<0.3	0.3–0.6	>0.6
0–6 mo	None	None	None
6 mo–3 y	0.25 mg/d[b]	None	None
3–6 y	0.50 mg/d	0.25 mg/d	None
6–16 y	1.0 mg/d	0.50 mg/d	None

[a] 1.0 parts per million (ppm) = 1 mg/L
[b] 2.2 mg of sodium fluoride contains 1 mg of fluoride ion

Careful assessment of all sources of dietary fluoride, including reconstituted infant formula and fluoridated toothpaste, is essential to avoid excessive intakes of fluoride, which can cause fluorosis and change the appearance of the teeth. The American Dental Association recommends that powdered or liquid concentrate infant formulas should be reconstituted using fluoridated drinking water; however, parents and health care providers should be aware of the risk for development of fluorosis.[39]

When fluorosis is a concern, the American Dental Association suggests that either ready-to-feed infant formula or powdered or liquid concentrate infant formula that has been reconstituted with fluoride-free or low-fluoride concentration water may be used.[39] The use of fluoridated toothpaste for children under the age of 6 years may increase the risk for developing fluorosis;

however, the benefits of using fluoridated toothpaste in terms of reduction of dental caries for those at high risk must be weighed against this potential increased risk.[40]

Calcium

Preschool and school-aged children and adolescents are increasingly at risk for inadequate intake of calcium because nondairy beverages, including soft drinks and fruit juices, are commonly consumed in place of milk.[20] In addition, other dairy foods, such as cheese or yogurt, which may be consumed as a substitute for milk are not necessarily fortified with vitamin D, thereby potentially limiting the body's ability to absorb and deposit calcium.[41]

Although hypocalcemia is rare, suboptimal calcium intake may result in poor bone mineralization, especially during adolescence when the majority of bone formation occurs.[41] The use of calcium supplements should be considered for children and adolescents who cannot or will not consume adequate dietary calcium to meet requirements; however, routine supplementation of healthy children with AI is not recommended.[20]

Vitamin B-12

Since the only sources of vitamin B-12 are animal foods, children and adolescents consuming a vegetarian diet or breastfed infants of vegetarian mothers may be at risk

Energy and
Nutrients

for deficiency. This is of greatest concern for children and adolescents following a vegan dietary pattern that excludes dairy products and eggs.

The same concern is applicable to breastfed infants of vegan mothers. The vitamin B-12 content of breastmilk is largely dependent on the mother's intake. Unless the mother is taking a vitamin B-12 supplement, breastfed infants of vegan mothers should receive 0.4 mcg vitamin B-12 daily from birth to 6 months, and 0.5 mcg vitamin B-12 daily beginning at 6 months and continuing until dietary intake of solid foods provides adequate vitamin B-12.[43]

References

1. Institute of Medicine. *Dietary Reference Intakes: Applications in Dietary Assessment.* Washington, DC: National Academies Press; 2000.

2. Institute of Medicine. DRI Tables and Application Reports. US Department of Agriculture website. www.nal.usda.gov /fnic/dri-tables-and-application-reports. Accessed May 22, 2019.

3. Institute of Medicine, Food and Nutrition Board, Panel on Macronutrients, Panel on the Definition of Dietary Fiber, Subcommittee on Upper Reference Levels of Nutrients, Subcommittee on Interpretation and Uses of Dietary Reference Intakes, Standing Committee on the Scientific Evaluation of Dietary Reference Intakes. *Dietary Reference Intakes for Energy, Carbohydrate, Fiber, Fat, Fatty Acids, Cholesterol, Protein, and Amino Acids.* Prepublication edition. Washington, DC: National Academies Press; 2005.

4. Weston SC, Murray P. Diet and nutrition. In: DeVore J, Shotton A, eds. *Academy of Nutrition and Dietetics Pocket Guide to Children with Special Health Care Needs: Nutrition Care Handbook.* Chicago, IL: Academy of Nutrition and Dietetics; 2012:22-75.

5. Green Corkins K, Whittenbrook W, eds. *Academy of Nutrition and Dietetics Pocket Guide to Children with Special Health Care and Nutritional Needs.* 2nd ed. Chicago, IL: Academy of Nutrition and Dietetics; in press.

6. World Health Organization. *Energy and Protein Requirements. Report of a Joint FAO/WHO/UNU Expert Consultation.* Technical Report Series 724. Geneva, Switzerland: World Health Organization; 1985.

7. Schofield WN. Predicting basal metabolic rate, new standards and review of previous work. *Hum Nutr Clin Nutr.* 1985;39C(suppl 1):S5-S42.

8. Sax HC, Souba WW. Nutritional goals and macronutrient requirements. In: *The ASPEN Nutrition Support Practice Manual.* Silver Spring, MD: ASPEN; 1998:1-5.

9. Page CP, Hardin TC, Melnik G, eds. *Nutritional Assessment and Support—A Primer.* 2nd ed. Baltimore, MD: Williams and Wilkins; 1994:32.

10. Barlow SE. Expert Committee recommendations regarding the prevention, assessment, and treatment of child and adolescent overweight and obesity: summary report. *Pediatrics.* 2007;120(suppl 4):S164-S192.

11. Lazzer S, Patrizi A, De Col A, Saezza A, Sartorio A. Prediction of basal metabolic rate in obese children and adolescents considering pubertal stages and anthropometric characteristics or body composition. *European J Clin Nutr.* 2014;68:695-699.

Energy and Nutrients

12. American Dietetic Association. Position of the American Dietetic Association: nutrient supplementation. *J Am Diet Assoc.* 2009;109:2073-2085.

13. Feeding the child. In: Kleinman RE, Greer FR, eds. *Pediatric Nutrition Handbook.* 7th ed. Elk Grove Village, IL: American Academy of Pediatrics; 2014:143-173.

14. Briefel R, Hanson C, Fox MK, Novak T, Ziegler P. Feeding Infants and Toddlers Study: do vitamin and mineral supplements contribute to nutrient adequacy or excess among US infants and toddlers? *J Am Diet Assoc.* 2006;106:S52-S65.

15. Committee on Fetus and Newborn, American Academy of Pediatrics. Controversies concerning vitamin K and the newborn. *Pediatrics.* 2003;112:191-192.

16. Sankar MJ, Chandrasekaran A, Kumar P, Thukral A, Agarwal R, Paul VK. Vitamin K prophylaxis for prevention of vitamin D deficiency bleeding: a systematic review. *J Perinatol.* 2016;36:S29-S34.

17. Weisberg P, Scanlon KS, Li R Cogswell ME. Nutritional rickets among children in the United States: review of cases reported between 1986 and 2003. *Am J Clin Nutr.* 2004;80(suppl):1697S-1705S.

18. Wagner CL, Greer FR; Section on Breastfeeding and Committee on Nutrition, American Academy of Pediatrics. Prevention of rickets and vitamin D deficiency in infants, children and adolescents. *Pediatrics.* 2008;122:1142-1152.

19. Misra M, Pacaud D, Petryk A, Collett-Solberg PA, Kappy M. Vitamin D deficiency in children and its management: review of current knowledge and recommendations. *Pediatrics.* 2008;122:398-417.

20.   Golden N, Abrams S, The Committee on Nutrition.
       Optimizing bone health in children and adolescents.
       Pediatrics. 2014;134:e1229-e1243.

21.   Prasanna N, Faridi MMA, Prerna B, Madhu SV. Oral
       supplementation of parturient mothers with vitamin D and
       its effect on 25OHD status of exclusively breastfed infants
       at 6 months of age: a double-blind randomized placebo
       controlled trial. *Breastfeeding Med.* 2017;12:621-628.

22.   Hollis BW, Wagner CL, Howard CR, et al. Maternal versus
       infant vitamin D supplementation during lactation: a
       randomized controlled trial. *Pediatrics.* 2015;136:625-634.

23.   Perrine CG, Sharma AJ, Jefferds MED, Serdula MK, Scanlon
       KS. Adherence to vitamin D recommendations among US
       infants. *Pediatrics.* 2010;125:627-632.

24.   Ahluwalia N, Herrick KA, Rossen LM, et al. Usual nutrient
       intakes of US infants and toddlers generally meet or exceed
       Dietary Reference Intakes: findings from NHANES 2009-
       2012. *Am J Clin Nutr.* 2016;104:1167-1174.

25.   Ginde AA, Sullivan AF, Mansbach JM, Camargo CA. Vitamin
       D insufficiency in pregnant and nonpregnant women of
       childbearing age in the United States. *Am J Obstet Gynecol.*
       2010;202:436.e1-e8.

26.   Johnson DD, Wagner CL, Hulsey TC, McNeil RB, Ebeling
       M, Hollis BW. Vitamin D deficiency and insufficiency is
       common during pregnancy. *Am J Perinatol.* 2011;28:7-12.

27.   Carvalho NF, Kenney RD, Carrington PH, Hall DE. Severe
       nutritional deficiencies in toddlers resulting from health
       food milk alternatives. *Pediatrics.* 2001;107:e46.

28. Baker RD, Greer FR, The Committee on Nutrition. Clinical report—diagnosis and prevention of iron deficiency and iron-deficiency anemia in infants and young children (0-3 years of age). *Pediatrics*. 2010;126:1040-1050.

29. Iron. In: Kleinman RE, Greer FR, eds. *Pediatric Nutrition Handbook*. 7th ed. Elk Grove Village, IL: American Academy of Pediatrics; 2014:449-466.

30. Friel JK, Aziz K, Andrews WL, Harding SV, Courage ML, Adams R. A double-masked, randomized controlled trial of iron supplementation in early infancy in healthy full-term infants. *J Pediatr*. 2003;143:582-586.

31. Ziegler EE, Nelson SE, Jeter JM. Iron supplementation of breastfed infants from an early stage. *Am J Clin Nutr*. 2009;89:525-532.

32. Cusick SE, Georgieff MK, Raghavendra R. Approaches for reducing the risk of early-life iron deficiency-induced brain dysfunction in children. *Nutrients*. 2018;10:227.

33. Centers for Disease Control and Prevention. Second National Report on Biochemical Indicators of Diet and Nutrition in the US Population. Washington, DC: Centers for Disease Control and Prevention; 2012. www.cdc.gov/nutritionreport. Accessed September 13, 2018.

34. Cogswell ME, Looker AC, Pfeiffer CM, et al. Assessment of iron deficiency in US preschool children and nonpregnant females of childbearing age: National Health and Nutrition Examination Survey 2003-2006. *Am J Clin Nutr*. 2009;89:1334-1342.

35. Nutrition and oral health. In: Kleinman RE, Greer FR, eds. *Pediatric Nutrition Handbook*. 7th ed. Elk Grove Village, IL: American Academy of Pediatrics; 2014:1167-1183.

36. US Department of Health and Human Services Federal Panel on Community Water Fluoridation. US Public Health Service recommendation for fluoride concentration in drinking water for the prevention of dental caries. *Public Health Rep.* 2015;130:318-331.

37. Tubert-Jeannin S, Auclair C, Amsallem E, et al. Fluoride supplements (tablets, drops, lozenges or chewing gums) for preventing dental caries in children. *Cochrane Database Syst Rev.* 2011;(12):CD007592.

38. Centers for Disease Control and Prevention. Recommendations for using fluoride to prevent and control dental caries in the United States. *MMWR Recomm Rep.* 2001;50(RR-14):1-42.

39. Berg J, Gerweck C, Hujoel PP, et al. Evidence-based clinical recommendations regarding fluoride intake from reconstituted infant formula and enamel fluorosis. *J Am Diet Assoc.* 2011;111:79-87.

40. Wong MCM, Glenny A, Tsang BWK, Lo ECM, Worthington HV, Marinho VCC. Topical fluoride as a cause of dental fluorosis in children. *Cochrane Database Syst Rev.* 2010;(1):CD007693.

41. Rizzoli R. Dairy products, yogurts and bone health. *Am J Clin Nutr.* 2014;99(suppl):1256S-1262S.

42. Calcium, Phosphorus, and Magnesium. In: Kleinman RE, ed. *Pediatric Nutrition Handbook.* 7th ed. Elk Grove Village, IL: American Academy of Pediatrics; 2014:435-448.

43. Institute of Medicine Standing Committee on the Scientific Evaluation of Dietary Reference Intakes and its Panel on Folate, Other B Vitamins, and Choline. *Dietary Reference Intakes for Thiamin, Riboflavin, Niacin, Vitamin B6, Folate, Vitamin B12, Pantothenic Acid, Biotin, and Choline.* Washington, DC: National Academies Press; 1998.

Continuing Professional Education

This third edition of *Academy of Nutrition Pocket Guide to Pediatric Nutrition Assessment* offers readers 5 hours of Continuing Professional Education (CPE) credit. Readers may earn credit by completing the interactive online quiz at the following link:

https://publications.webauthor.com/pg_to_ped _nutr_asses_3e

Index

Page number followed by *t* indicates table, and page number followed by *b* indicates box.

Page numbers followed by *t* indicate tables, and page numbers followed by *b* indicate boxes.